# THE BOOK OF LOVE

T.M.

## *FORTHCOMING*

*The Book of LOVE* is one-half of a two book effort.
This nonfiction work is a description of the nature of love
and how love grows and develops.

The companion volume is a novel called *The Power of Love*,
and through it one can experience directly
the emotions involved in a great love –
and learn just what it is
that so many are foolishly throwing away today
without the slightest hesitation.

## *ALSO BY JAMES R. MESSENGER*

### Books

*EXCUSE ME, PLEASE, BUT I'D LIKE MY GOVERNMENT BACK*

*THE DEATH OF THE AMERICAN TELEPHONE & TELEGRAPH COMPANY – HOW "MA BELL" DIED GIVING BIRTH TO THE INFORMATION AGE*

### Films

"OF TIME, TOMBS AND TREASURE:
The Treasures of Tutankhamun"
Academy Award® Nomination - Best Documentary Short Subject

"KORYO CELADON"
Academy Award Nomination - Best Documentary Short Subject

"THE TAJ MAHAL"
National EMMY® - Best Documentary
National EMMY - Best Cinematography

"CARRY THE FIRE: The Story of the 1984 Olympic Torch Relay"

### Video

"DEFINING THE INFORMATION AGE"

# THE BOOK OF LOVE

T.M.

*The Guidebook*
*For Anyone*
*Who Ever Wanted To Be*
*In Love*

**James R. Messenger**

THE ALEXANDER PRESS LLC
*Marietta, Georgia*

Books like no others.™

THE ALEXANDER PRESS LLC
*Fine Quality Printing & Publishing*
www.thealexanderpress.com
Post Office Box 681444
Marietta, Georgia 30068

Hardback ISBN 978-0-914695-02-8
Paperback ISBN 978-0-914695-03-5

Library of Congress Control Number: 2008906620



*Please Take a Moment to Read*

This book is a personal essay on the nature of love as I have known it. *The Book of Love* is sold with the understanding that neither the publisher nor the author is engaged in rendering relationship counseling, psychological assistance, or any other professional service. If expert assistance is required to help you with the circumstances of your life, the services of a competent professional should be sought.

*Quantity book discounts are available to schools, religious organizations, and other appropriate non-profits teaching "Love Education."*

*The emblem of The Alexander Press LLC is a portrait of Alexander the Great portrayed as Heracles, with a lion's mane headdress, on a tetradrachm from the royal mint of Amphipolis, circa 336-323 B.C.*

*The Alexander Press LLC logo was designed by Kevin C. Drexler.*

*Printed on archival quality paper.*

*For You,*

*And for anyone who has ever wanted to know love.*

# THE BOOK OF LOVE

T.M.

# CONTENTS

There was a boy,
A very strange, enchanted boy.
They say he came from very far, very far,
Over land and sea.
A little shy,
And sad of eye,
But very wise was he.
And then one day,
One magic day, he passed my way,
And we spoke of many things,
Fools and kings,
And this he said to me:
"The greatest thing
You'll ever learn
Is just to love
And be loved
In return."

– "*Nature Boy*"
Eden Abhez

# INTRODUCTION

♥ This book was written for one simple reason: From what I can perceive today, it appears that people everywhere have come to believe that love does not really exist. This is something I find truly tragic.

People will deny they believe such a thing. They will state immediately that, of course, they believe love is real. But if you look at the panorama of life before us – the average life of a marriage is now two years; most children are growing up in one-parent households; and, films, TV, books, magazines, music, and advertising all suggest that casual sex is all there is to love – one cannot help but come to the conclusion that "something is not quite right with this picture." The evidence suggests that today people believe almost anything but that love is real.

So what I wish to provide with this little book is something completely counter to almost all contemporary thinking on the subject of love. This book is designed to provide an understanding of the true nature of love: What it is; how it grows and develops; and how to keep it for all of your life.

What is my expertise for having a say on this subject? I am not a psychologist or a marriage counselor or a sociologist or any other kind of professional "expert" on the subject. And I certainly don't pretend to take the place of those important advisers whom,

I am sure, do yeoman's duty in trying to aid people in gaining and holding love in these complex and difficult times.

What I am is a man who has had the extraordinary good fortune to know, not just love, but monumental love in my life. And what I intend to do is to describe what I learned from standing on that mountaintop.

Love, I can say from personal experience, is very real. And it is the single most extraordinary thing a human being can ever experience. When I look about me and see how many people will pass through this life and world and will never know love, it pains me to a degree I almost cannot bear. So I wrote this book in response to that pain. In some small way, I hope I can make a difference in just a few lives, so that at least that many more human beings will know the glory of love.

Perhaps you will be one of them.

Do I have a message with this book? Yes, indeed. You actually should know it already. If you read the poem – actually song lyrics – by Eden Abhez, then you have read my message, which is contained in the simplest, but wisest, words you will ever come across:

"The greatest thing
You'll ever learn
Is just to love
And be loved in return."

Anything else I have to say is simply additional support for that most wondrous expression.

# 1. SOME HISTORICAL PERSPECTIVE

♥ Love has been a constant theme in human affairs over nearly all time. It is natural that the relationship between men and women would be of interest to our species. But there has been something more to this interest between women and men than mere curiosity about mating and bonding behaviors for survival of our species.

The discovery – as depicted in virtually all of the arts – of the existence and power of love and the behaviors that men and women will exhibit – both good and bad – in an attempt to possess it, speaks to the fact that there must be some truth to the reality of love, or else humans would not have put so much labor into recording it. And, just as important, all of these efforts document that love is an emotional state much to be desired.

History records many such human stories: Anthony and Cleopatra, Abelard and Heloise, Napoleon and Josephine, the Duke and Duchesse of Windsor, Hank and Audrey Williams, F. Scott and Zelda Fitzgerald, Sara and Gerald Murphy, Paul Newman and Joanne Woodward, and the list goes on – past and present.

So why does it seem, in our day and age, that love is so difficult to find, and why does it appear to so many of us that men and women have somehow evolved into separate species whose only commonality is the need for the occasional and casual sexual release and brief bondings so that children might be created to carry the species on?

There are actually very complex reasons for the evolution of human society – some created by accident, others by intention – but for our purposes the main result of current historical forces is that these changes in our society have brought about almost complete distrust between men and women today. And since absolute trust between women and men, as we shall soon see, is the only possible foundation for real and true love, it now appears quite reasonable to the modern mind to conclude that love does not, in fact, exist, but is merely a beautiful poetic fiction to glamorize the more animalistic side of human sexuality. Love, so many now actually believe, is nothing more or nothing less than a nice idea.

The result of this belief is a great deal of loneliness, of people living out their lives separately instead of together – even when married and living in the same household – with the feeling of a constant ache, a constant void that cannot be filled, being the hint that there MUST be something more than merely passing through this life and moving on.

Well, there is more. And if you can understand what you're looking for – you'd be amazed at how many people, when confronted with the possibility for love and real romance, find there is good reason for pushing it out of their lives as "abnormal" behavior – love is still there for the taking.

# 2. WHY MOST GREAT STORIES ARE ABOUT LOVE

♥ Anyone who has known real love doesn't need to read this chapter – such lucky people don't need an explanation for the chapter title. And, like the beautiful love story in the motion picture "The Notebook," the power of real love – however long or brief its possession may be – is a blessing that one can turn to for a lifetime.

Though the pattern love takes within any life which encounters it remains relatively constant in the manner it comes into being and evolves – though any couple who's ever discovered the reality of love is sure in their conclusion that the love they know is unique to all time – it is the fact that most people are left to discover love accidentally, rather than having any skills or expectations in how to find it, that leaves most of the world destitute of real love.

Ironically, the greatest writers and artists and musicians have tried their best to capture the essence of love, to convey hints as to how to recognize it when one sees it. For instance, what makes William Shakespeare's sonnets the most extraordinary poems ever written is that – through the magic of words – Shakespeare captured the reality of a great love to the degree that one feels one is a participant in this great flood of emotion.

After reading the "Sonnets," it is typical for people to wonder: "What if someone had loved ME that much and was able to tell me how they truly felt in loving me?" The same can be true after hearing remarkable pieces of music, with the extraordinary songs "I Have a Love" and "One Hand, One Heart" from "West Side Story;" or Frank Loesser's "My Heart Is So Full of You" from "Most Happy Fella;" or the tragic "Un Bel Di" ("One Beautiful Day") from Puccini's opera "Madame Butterfly" all trying to capture the sheer richness and depth of feeling that is the essential nature of love.

Once known, real love simply can't be forgotten. Matter of fact, love transforms people completely into a person they weren't before, something most cannot believe possible until it happens. Once through that doorway, things are never the same again.

Interestingly enough, love stories can actually be told in many different ways. One of the most beautiful love stories is a "story" made out of stone. Anyone who has ever had an opportunity to visit the Taj Mahal cannot doubt that this extraordinary building made of both marble and sky is the testimony to a truly monumental love.

Indeed, in my estimation, and stemming from my personal experience, I believe that the greatest sight on this planet is Taj Mahal by the light of a full moon. In the gentle moonlight, the building becomes exquisitely feminine. It appears before one transformed – having turned into a soft, diaphanous image so delicate that one goes through periodic panics while gazing upon it for fear that a breeze might stir up and blow this fragile, floating monument to love completely away. And the thought of Taj Mahal being no more is simply unbearable to those who have been captured by its seductive beauty.

The power of the building is such that I can remember that when I saw it for the very first time, I could either look at the tour guide and listen to the history of Taj Mahal, or I could let my eyes drift over to the building and the man's voice would simply fade away into nothing as the building poured emotion towards me. And consider that if this is the way a complete stranger feels, what must it have been like to have been inside that monumental love?

***Many stories, one story***

Because of its power, the story of love is passed from one generation to the next by those who have known it, so that it might not be forgotten. And most artists and writers want it to be known that love is worth absolutely everything when one finds it – Shakespeare's"Romeo and Juliet;" Bizet's opera "Carmen," the novels and movies of *The Thornbirds* and *Gone With the Wind* being just a few examples – and the list goes on and on and on in every nation and in every tongue around the world, for the phenomenon is worldwide.

When one has the extraordinary good fortune to walk through the doorway to love, everything – absolutely everything – changes to a degree most cannot even comprehend as being possible. And each time new lovers make the "find," the desire to share and celebrate this wondrous experience keeps the knowledge of love alive.

The power of love is of such magnitude that there has never been a time when discoverers have ever concluded that there might be some greater subject in the world for literature, art, music, or whatever other means might be available to help tell the tale. Among human beings, there is simply no other experience – wealth, fame, or any of the other worldly goals that people might pursue or possess – that comes anywhere close to the shimmering experience of real love.

If it makes anyone feel better, it is also true that until one experiences love, one has no way of judging the reality of it. Love, when achieved, comes as the most dazzling surprise to everyone who gets there. Even if you are a hopeless Romantic, no matter how much you have fantasized about it, no matter how high your expectations, no matter how you imagined love might be – you will be wrong. And love will be better and more amazing than anything you could have projected or hoped for.

And that's precisely why one needs to learn how to get to love and how to keep it.

# 3. IS LOVE WORTH FIGHTING FOR?

♥ In a word, "Yes." How can one not believe that something that has proven the most precious thing humans can possess, and which is simply beyond price – no amount of money being able to buy it – is not worth pursuing? Add to that the amazing fact that love is something virtually anyone of any status or rank might one day have, which is an astounding concept in a world currently driven only by money or "15 minutes of fame," where most feel left out and disenfranchised. When our lives seem so often circumscribed today, love is one of the last standards to bear that can bring real results in terms of true human happiness.

However, as is also true today, in this day and age, the commitment one must make to find love can be an uphill battle all the way. The obstacles can be virtually overwhelming. For instance, subtle changes have taken place in society, at least American society, that make it very difficult for people looking for a mate to even meet. The explosion of dating services, newspaper matchmaking advertisements, Internet sites, etc., all speak to this difficulty.

And lessons in civil and social behavior between the sexes, such as ballroom dancing – a wonderful activity that used to allow young people to meet and talk with the opposite sex on a more intimate basis as a positive means of learning about one another – have all but been abandoned.

The creation of fear amongst people as a trend among popular culture – for instance, the bizarre simultaneous encouragement and revilement by the news media of the phenomenon of "stalking" being one remarkable example – has made people in general very hesitant and mistrustful. In another example, television and films "instruct" us on a daily basis that the highest American values are apparently money, the desire to murder one another, and raw, casual sex – with love nowhere to be seen amongst those priorities.

And what about the work place? "Sexual harassment" cases – accusations against one another – have been "fashionable" for quite some time, and, sadly, the increasingly casual application of this legal weapon has created a world of fear between the sexes: One misstep, should one find someone one is interested in getting to know at work, and one is out on the street and out of a job.

There is also another message promoted by the huge corporate bureaucracies today, which is extremely detrimental to the growth and development of love. Love is all about emotion, deep feelings, about passion. Bureaucracies, especially large-scale bureaucracies such as now exist in global enterprises, are based upon the concept of "objective control." A human being who exhibits any kind of passion (with some leeway allowed for sports enthusiasts, since sports are believed to help drive the competitive spirit) is suspect. Such people are viewed as likely to spin "out of control," and careers can often end when any kind of real emotion is shown.

The emphasis upon this pattern of behavior has caused many people to develop a revulsion for passion, even outside of work hours. For instance, in direct contrast to traditional notions of love and attracting a mate, many women today are actually offended by men who give them presents, or write them letters, or engage in any of the traditional wooing practices. To do such is not viewed as showing one's interest, but as "coming on too strong."

Some women today – perhaps this is true of men, too; I cannot say – are even offended by standard "getting to know you" questions such as "What do you do for fun?"; "Do you have a favorite movie?"; "Do you enjoy travel?"; etc. Indeed, I had an experience with one woman who said she felt like men were "giving her the third degree" by asking such questions and were "prying into her life." To this person, there were only two possible subjects for discussion – her work and her favorite baseball team. She believed "getting to know someone" meant sitting in silence and simply staring at each other, and that some sort of osmosis of the spirits would take place by doing so. When one considers that true love is mostly about real, rich, human communications, consider what this kind of attitude achieves – and what changes must have occurred within a society where a human being would actually have come to believe a "relationship" to consist of nothing more than merely sitting in silence with another human being?

In addition, look at the mixed messages of advertising – the use of pornographic images of both women and men are now used on a daily basis and "sold" as the image of the "good life:" Lust. Sex. Constant sexual heat.

But what happens when people attempt to act upon that daily instruction and role model? Such behavior suddenly becomes taboo in real life and punishment can be swift and sure. And are we to believe that the thousands of teenage unwed mothers that have resulted from "doing as they were told" by our communications media such as TV and movies and ending up in a state of constant struggle is ***not*** a form of punishment?

Another phenomenon of our time is the growth of "man-bashing." While serving as a source of great entertainment on the part of many women, this practice has resulted in added distrust and distance, since the way propaganda works is that such "humor" invariably becomes "fact" after a while – rather than remaining as a mere form of humor – due to the sheer repetition of it.

## TWO SONNETS IN A BOOK STORE

### I. A Woman to a Man

The unknown came to shine for me today,
When all I wished was Shakespeare's sonnets found.
You took the time to seek for me and stayed,
When easy search had run upon dry ground.
Your patience gave me time enough to stare
At you, at what God's handiwork had wrought.
Such manly beauty God could not have dared,
And knowing so, I never would have sought.
But living, breathing, moving, I beheld,
This fairest sight that took my breath from me.
And, suddenly, I found myself in Hell,
With mute words crying out to Destiny:
        "If there is any justice to one's Fate,
        Then tell me now that I have found my mate!!"

## II. A Man to a Woman

**Don't turn** me down from first and shocked surprise,
At finding a man in whom love's still awake,
In learning there are those who, through the eyes,
Still see the upward way to Heaven's gate.
Your face, your voice, your spirit strong,
Your manner kind and good,
Spoke to my heart – I thought – in song,
That made me hope you would
Lift up your eyes to look at me
Beyond the skeptic's gaze,
And see that there's a chance to be
In love for all your days.
So, please, *before* you shut your heart,
Consider well these words of art.

JAMES R. MESSENGER

As a result, women engaging in this activity – without even realizing it – begin to look at men far differently and can readily begin making cynical interpretations of a man's behavior that has no basis in fact, but every basis in the jaundiced view developed towards men through man-bashing.

So what are the substitutes being offered to people in lieu of role models of love, which is where our attention *should* be focused? Today's human ideals typically projected are:

- Casual, uncommitted sex
- The importance of money and material goods
- Selfishness as a high value
- Vicarious thrills via movies, TV, novels, magazines, the Internet, etc.

In short: Emptiness.

And in terms of our spiritual and philosophical needs today, what are we really being offered? For instance, does anyone truly believe in the sentiments of the "Declaration of Independence" anymore, i.e. do we really believe and treat each other as equal Citizens? Do we have a great national goal that inspires us to work as one nation? Do the businesses we work for promote a common vision in which all employees can believe?

I think not. The closest thing we have today in America that resembles anything like a true national event is the Super Bowl, where huge amounts of guilt are applied to ensure the watching of what is usually one of the great "yawners" of football each year, ordinarily so boring that the TV commercials have become the substitute topic for discussion. Can one really believe in chips and dip and football as a national belief system, particularly when what is typically served up is sales hype and not a common inspiration regarding human excellence? Can such emptiness inspire people to get up each day to go to work?

And are we being given real substance from our religions? That's a personal answer for each of us, but one must wonder when so many religions are spending a great deal of time promoting – not love – but hatred for people who are different from them and who might engage in practices they don't happen to like. Is this really the kind of "food for the soul" we need?

Because it is part of being human to have a need to believe and participate in something larger than oneself, spiritual emptiness of the forms described above actually have a very direct impact on how people see the world and each other. In sum, because we no longer perceive a common bond, either in public or at work, a great deal of coldness, emptiness, and meaninglessness has become the order of the day, something that impacts almost every aspect of our lives. And as we get colder towards one another, it becomes even harder to break through to love.

As just one example, as many women can attest, one of the greatest roadblocks to real intimacy and moving to the level of emotion known as love is a complete inability for many men to say the three most difficult words in the English language: "I love you." The difficulties that lie behind this phrase are, of course, quite complex for many people. But some observations can still be made.

For instance, the apparent admission of weakness that this phrase implies to many men in saying they depend upon a woman is completely alien to the tough guy, stand-alone hero image that men are asked to adhere to in our Western society. Thus, one can immediately understand the role model of James Bond and others like him who "take" sex from women without commitment and are admired as heroes and "real men." No weakness shown there.

Plus to others, saying "I love you" is like suddenly entering into a woman's world, which is a place that remains very mysterious and alarming to many men, with the possibility that something unpredictable and uncontrollable might happen. Many men, because the greatest need of men is for respect, cannot abide the idea of being embarrassed or being held up to ridicule, so it can be an easy conclusion that it is safer to stay as far away from this potential danger as possible. And, thus for so many, love ends – or, really, never begins – because it seems impossible to cross this line.

The net result of all these forces upon our hearts and minds has been to destroy the single most important value that is the ONLY foundation for love – trust.

Trust is, of course, based upon honesty. And if one looks around one, how much real honesty does one now see? On the part of government? On the part of business? On the part of people's daily behavior?

Who can one trust? How can one allow oneself to become vulnerable enough to trust another fully? That has now become the crux of the modern dilemma of love.

Today, a large number of people never can get past answering those questions. And, thus, they never encounter real love, which, in turn, leads them to conclude there is no such thing as love. It simply does not exist. It cannot exist. And, on that basis, a consensus has been achieved in our time that love is dead, perhaps never existed, or is merely a fiction of someone's imagination. And, so many – and it hurts to say, perhaps even most – live lives of quiet desperation, with mere companionship and a shattered illusion about the existence of love.

But I'm telling you – love isn't dead. It's alive and well. You just need to know how to get to it.

# 4. WHY DON'T WE TEACH OUR CHILDREN ABOUT LOVE?

♥ I obviously cannot speak for other cultures, but in the United States – as many from outside our borders have observed over the years – Americans have the most peculiar and contradictory hang-ups about sex and love. For instance, we as a people see no particular problem with sex being used aggressively to sell virtually any kind of product – practically naked women and men pant before our very eyes in the heat of sexual passion on a daily basis suggesting that this or that product will provide what those models possess. In films and even in our very homes on TV, people now regularly copulate before our eyes. Lurid romance novels sell like gangbusters and are now staples of bestseller lists. Magazines and newspapers regularly report the details of the sexual life of actors and actresses and other celebrities. In short, the American people are swimming in a sea of sex.

One would think that if this much sex in our lives is now a "normal" environment, most parents would not have much trouble talking about sex and love with their children. But many – if perhaps not most – parents have a big problem with that discussion. And they also possess an awful lot of excuses to avoid the subject.

For instance, in my own family, my entire sex education consisted of being furtively shown a book on how babies are created – and that was the end of it. There were no other discussions. There was an awful lot of frowning that indicated most anything to do with sex was considered wrong and "dirty." But the words "love" or "sex" were never even mentioned in my household.

When I raised this issue in adulthood, the answer given to me was that my father's parents never talked to him about sex, so, therefore, he wasn't going to discuss it either. And that apparently was considered reason enough for leaving a child completely on his own to figure out what was happening to him during one of the monumental stages of his development (and this was true for my sister and brother as well).

What's particularly sad is that this is not any kind of unusual story, but more towards the norm – at least for the entire generation in which I grew up. And it apparently continues to a large degree today, at least from the anecdotal comments I've heard, with so many young people still developing their ideas about appropriate sexual/love behavior by watching their peers – or even worse, by watching films and TV, studying advertising messages, listening to music with sexually oriented lyrics, etc.

The subject of sex education – not to mention love education – is so emotionally charged, that it remains generally non-existent in schools, and is something often actively fought when proposed as a school subject. Many parents are terrified that their children might "get ideas" and become sexually active. But, they also typically fail to replace such education when taken from the schools with "home schooling." It just returns to being an unmentioned subject, so any form of reasonable and objective knowledge that might give a sensible basis for young people to think about their changing bodies and minds is successfully avoided.

It is, of course, the emotionally charged nature of sex and love that is the crux of the problem. In dealing with matters of sex, parents are touching upon the deepest emotions of the human creature. And when so many of us are "walking wounded" ourselves, having had no such education, and with a fair number of marriages being flawed matches having very little to do with love, it makes sex and love education all the more difficult. One may safely assume there's a reason the average marriage is now only two years in length and that more than 50 percent of all marriages end in divorce.

Those parents who do talk to their children about sex and the role it plays in love are to be applauded. And there are some church groups and other family organizations that try to fulfill this task, but, sadly, too often with rather uneven results, sometimes admirably, and sometimes selling political propaganda about sexuality in substitution for solid knowledge. But in the main, as far as I have been able to tell, most parents spend their time "hoping" their children will simply absorb by osmosis the things they see in their parents' marriage as a role model for love.

It is rather astounding that Humankind has come so far down the line time-wise in history, yet has never really learned how to deal with one of the most important aspects of human existence – the finding and nurturing of love. Indeed, as I observed earlier, we have even created an environment where many people – despite the fact that so much of what we see around us is talk about "love, sex, and relationships" – no longer believe that love is even real.

But, as I'll state again, love IS real, and I believe the ultimate human prize. And, if one is able to achieve monumental love, one can readily recognize that such an achievement is the greatest accomplishment Humans can strive for... All the armies that ever marched, all the ships that ever sailed, all the deeds that were ever done, cannot measure up to the riches of true love.

And we have even apparently forgotten – it used to be expressed in what would now be considered a "chauvinist male" cliché that "behind every successful man is a good woman" – that it is far easier to accomplish great things in any field or occupation when one is standing on the foundation of and moving through life with the support of a great love.

It is my estimation that if our society is to improve itself so that we can advance to a new level of human existence, it seems rather reasonable that a good way to do that would be to begin the process of educating our children in the ways of love.

Note that I did not say "the ways of sex."

Though the terms "sex" and "love" are used completely interchangeably today, they are not the same thing at all. And to my mind, it is far more important to teach the ways of love than the ways of sex, for the ways of love are far more important if one is to achieve true intimacy and an environment that will enable love to last a lifetime. Sex happens to be only one means to that end.

And that, of course, brings us back to what this book is all about. You'll come to understand as you read further, that "getting to love" is the point. If you want your children to know – or if you want to know yourself – what it takes to get to love, read on.

In the years to come, I would like to think there will be many books far more sophisticated than this one to help move us to a new and happier level of human existence. But for a first venture into new and uncharted territory, I believe you'll find this work sufficient to make the scales fall from the eyes of anyone who takes this journey to the end destination, whereby he or she can begin to comprehend what love is really about.

# 5. TRUST – THE ONE AND ONLY FOUNDATION FOR LOVE

♥ Trust. This one word tells the tale of why so many marriages today wind up on the rocks. Lack of trust is the single greatest blockade to people ever getting to love.

Trust is a difficult subject to deal with in reality. That's because we've created a society in which "distrust" has been sold as the mode "sharp and intelligent" people should operate in. We are advised that "everyone is working an angle," everyone is "looking out for #1," and anyone naïve enough to trust another person is a fool.

And those messages are regularly confirmed for us: For instance, the core staple of TV is ultimate distrust – murder. Everyone is angry. Everyone is full of rage. Everyone needs to get even. Everyone needs to run people over to become a success. Everyone is trying to score a quick "lay." No one follows the old belief that used to be a fundamental American value – to trust someone until proven otherwise.

The degree of that distrust, though it is gradually becoming more uniform over time, does vary from one part of America to another. For instance, I recall moving back to the South after living in the Northeast for ten years and finding myself suspicious of every sales clerk, simply because he or she spoke to me, something that I no longer experienced where I previously had lived. They were doing so, of course, out of politeness, something I hadn't seen in years, having lived in a culture that had become so abrasive, it was considered taboo to simply say "Good morning" to anyone, for such would be viewed as a sign of weakness.

As another example of the trends within our society, it also seems to matter very little to almost anyone that the desensitizing example of murder on TV has become a television staple now provided as an example of "normal" human behavior virtually every night of the week. This lazy method of TV production – despite the cries of the networks that "it's only harmless TV" – has yielded many behaviors that have taken a heavy toll on American life: Young people who go ahead and commit murder because it's "okay" to do so on TV, thereby ruining their lives; people who develop a paranoid sense that they "can't trust anyone anymore," etc.

As still another example, we're now repeatedly living the experience of our top leaders in politics, religion, business, education, etc., possessing feet of clay, rather than being role models of great vision and character to inspire a nation. A trusting environment simply appears to be non-existent in the United States today.

So with distrust now being the "norm," it's very difficult to give even a single reason why one should trust another human being. But there is one good reason to learn to trust: It's the one and only way you're ever going to get to love. Without that foundation, it simply ain't ever gonna happen, to use really down to earth language. That really is a basic truth of the Universe.

As an example, I continue to be haunted by the final image of the film "I Love Trouble," which starred Julia Roberts and Nick Nolte as two competing reporters who wind up "falling in love" and getting married. During the entire film the pair has lied to each other and cheated on one another in competing over writing a newspaper story they had supposedly agreed to "partner" on. In the film's final scene, the two rivals have married and make a promise to "shoot straight" with one another. But each has fingers and feet crossed to break the vow.

This might have made a "cute and clever" ending to the film, but predict the future of that marriage. Just how long do you think a relationship based upon lies will last? "I Love Trouble" was clearly the right title for that movie, for that will be the "theme" of such a marriage.

It should also be noted that when it comes to lying, there are many ways people can lie. They can simply do it outright. They can do it by leaving out parts of stories. They can do it by keeping a part of themselves private and secret. These latter kinds of liars often don't believe they're lying. They can feel they're just handling truth "carefully." But it's hard to imagine when two people combine to become one that there can be much justification or circumstances for withholding critical information from one's spouse. If two-become-one in marriage, they've thrown their lot in together and should move through the world that way. Any other method is for two people to remain two, and that's not a marriage. And it's certainly not love.

This is not to suggest that brutal truth be hurled at everything. Common decency says that part of the nature of a relationship is caring for one another's feelings. What I am suggesting is that when it comes to the central issues of a love, anything less than truth and trust is simply driving in a wedge that will almost invariably divide two people in the end.

The kind of trust one must establish for love is readily demonstrated by a common team building activity used by many companies and organizations. (Please *don't* try this exercise without professional supervision.) The exercise is for an individual to stand on a wall about four feet high facing backwards.

The person spreads out his or her arms and then simply falls backwards to be caught by the team of people standing behind them. Many find this – quite rightly – very difficult to do. Trust is believing that there is someone behind you, someone who will always catch you to break your fall and keep you from hurting yourself. Until one does this exercise, it's a bit hard to understand just how difficult trusting can be when you're going to blindly fall backwards and simply trust that someone will be there. But that is precisely how trust operates in true love: "Two become one," and, in turn, support one another as though they were one, with one set of common interests.

The described experience is, of course, a group exercise, with the rest of the team standing below to cushion the fall. But this kind of trust characterizes precisely what two individuals achieve who are in love. There is simply no division between the two. One doesn't have to always be looking over one's shoulder, as is suggested is "reality" by almost all communications media today. Life is a confident matter, because you look to one another and don't need anyone else.

And the exercise also depicts another aspect of falling in love. Look at the expression we use to describe the process of coming together in love. We say "falling in love." Have you ever thought about why people would use such an expression?

Most people are caught off guard when real love begins to happen. That's because it's not what one expects at all, and there's really no way to prepare for the feeling. The sensation is entirely like two people are falling into one another – and you are. And you can really only "let go" completely and fall – which you must do to reach love – if you trust the other person. If you can't let yourself fall, if you pull yourself up short out of fear or lack of trust, you break the link and never get to love. And many are the people who have destroyed their possibility for love right at the start from such fear.

The sense of falling is so complete that a common statement by those who pull themselves out of the situation is "I don't like to lose control." American culture is so control-bound in our work, in our expectation that people will follow the "Rulebook of Life" – which everyone is supposed to know by instinct – that ever-so-many people won't let themselves know love, because they have no idea where these feelings of "falling" might be taking them, and they have no concepts whatsoever as to how to guide the emotions.

The underlying trust between two lovers must be complete because love is also not one thing. It's a continuously evolving journey that gets richer with each passing day and year. And unless one is grounded in trust in one another, ready and prepared to support each other as each evolution and change comes, at some point it will be as if that river of love becomes dammed and love will cease to be, because one can simply go no further.

The best way to get to that trust in this day and age is to take the time to get to know one another: See how your interests match. Go experience each other's life by trying out something each of you like but the other has never tried. Take the time to talk – over coffee, over lunch, over dinner – use any excuse. Why? Because the glue of trust is communication.

And if you failed to hear me say that, listen again: "The glue of trust is communication." If you fail to learn that one lesson, then you will fail at trust, and it won't matter whatever else you do – whether it be gifts or vacations together or whatever – you'll be doomed to failure and will never keep love alive.

How truly important are trust and truth? In my personal life, I have observed only one rule that never fails me: the first time someone deliberately lies to me, that relationship is done, for he or she can never be fully trusted again after that. That may sound severe, but I am actually a very flexible person who will tolerate a great deal in my life in terms of human behavior, because I know most situations between people can be fixed. But my one rule about lying has proven sure and true. With the exception of something silly like a surprise birthday party, there really is no condition between people in love where lying is ever a legitimate act. NEVER.

The moment a lie happens between lovers and one becomes aware of it, one will forever be looking over one's shoulder in doubt. And that little seed never fails to grow when planted. And when one comes to the conclusion that one can no longer risk "falling backwards blindly" because there's no longer any assurance he or she will be caught, love is as good as dead.

Many will view my "slow down the trip to the bedroom" attitude, and "get to know one another to establish strong communications" old-fashioned and naïve. After all, "everyone knows" sophisticated people today are "fully responsible" and enjoy sexual pleasure whenever they like. And perhaps that's true. But were we talking about sex? We were talking about love, and that is something as different from sex as night is from day.

There is also remarkable peer pressure on people today to "score" in order to show they're hip, attractive, and, most important, desirable. Such used to be a phenomenon exhibited almost exclusively by men to demonstrate their virility. But, now, many women can't be seen as "liberated" unless they're bed hopping, which is a rather amazing attitude in the era of AIDS.

And one should remember this: The intimate exercise of one's genitals in an intimate situation is not trust, though someone wanting you to do this will most assuredly say it is. The expression "one night stand" tells the tale of that form of "trust."

The difference I'm trying to depict is about creating a foundation for love that can lead to very fulfilling sex, versus merely finding a means to have sex. Since most people confuse the two, and the fact that so many people no longer believe love really exists, the typical outcome of the latter approach can readily be predicted.

And if you only pursue that latter path, the odds are that you'll actually have a good chance of eventually marrying someone who will remain pretty much a stranger for the rest of your life, unless a small miracle happens, as it will from time to time, where people find trust and love by luck after they wed.

The choice, ladies and gentlemen, will, of course, be yours. And, as many have found – shocking as this may seem – sex can tend to wear thin over time, but love does not. Love grows in strength and power, lifting one up all one's life, and then when you add in sex – WHOA!

Think about it. Trust is the key. There isn't any other foundation for love. There isn't. I'm sorry. Fool yourself all you want to the contrary. You'll always come up short in the end if you follow any other course.

Trust is it. Period. Paragraph.

♥

# 6. HOW DOES LOVE GROW AND DEVELOP?

♥ As proven by the millions of words that have been written, the thousands of songs that have been composed and sung, the endless paintings that have tried to capture the emotions of love, the many films and plays that have been made to tell the tale, love is a very complex subject.

Some claim love is a unique psychological experience. Some claim it is many things going by the same name. There is great confusion and endless difficulty in getting to the heart of the subject. So how does one get one's hands around the subject of love to provide any real meaning?

Well, here's my approach: What I intend to provide for you is a model of love's growth and development that will move from first stages up to the state of monumental love. And I will surround this with observations I have made along the way as I traveled that route myself. This is a very personal model – one that I believe holds true for most people – but it is not a scientific claim I'm making that's been proven as documented fact. It is – and should remain so in your mind – my personal witness to the experience of love as I lived it, and as I have observed it in others.

Those who have managed to achieve true love will, I believe, recognize readily what I say. And those who have never yet gotten to love will find this model to be a very useful tool for understanding what to expect and what to seek. It is, I believe, exactly what is missing in our society today as people everywhere try and "guess" their way to love – and, likewise, also "guess" their way forward in the development of love once they have found it. And just as a road map is not geography itself, but a useful tool for getting to one's destination, so, too, you will find the "road map" I provide extremely useful whether your "highway" to love follows this exact model or not.

But, first, it's important to ask this question: Why would anyone even want to be in love? The evidence presented today by all avenues of communication suggests that the disadvantages now outweigh the advantages. According to all of these sources, we need to settle for temporary "sexual release" and to forget about the rest. Or so we have come to believe through endless repetition of those messages.

If one will look at merely the surface of things today – not even citing statistical studies – one can see in many of one's friends that the amount of work and energy people must put into just dating is draining; that the constant ache that is loneliness can be nearly completely debilitating to people at times in terms of their working effectiveness – and, in not a few cases – can lead to alcoholism and other problems; that the struggle of managing a one-parent household is something very hard and stressful; and the list goes on and on. Are we really so sure that "independence" is worth such a price? Is it really more trouble to be in love than it is to live a "free and easy" life where one goes home to an empty apartment or house filled with silence and little human comfort?

With those questions in mind, let's look at a typical model of the evolution of love and what it takes to grow and maintain it.

***It all begins in childhood***

First, the ability to love – which is tied so closely with the ability to trust – really begins, as psychologists will tell you, in infancy. Were you held a lot as a child? Did you learn early the importance of touch and to become relaxed in exhibiting this behavior as a natural behavior?

Touch is one of the very first communications media we learn to use. Those who think only words communicate are in error. There is a whole range of ways that people communicate with one another – body language, touch, the way we dress, etc. – all giving signals to others about the way we feel about ourselves as well as others.

Those who come from cold and formal families – surprise!! – tend to be cold and formal in their own actions, feeling other types of behaviors are "unnatural." Those who come from families where nudity was frowned upon in their youth, again, tend to equate shame with the naked body, and feel very uncomfortable around people who tend to be more casual about nakedness.

In short, so much of what one brings to the table when it comes to love is baggage we have carried along with us for all of our life. And this emotional baggage colors the interpretation we have when we try to understand what love is.

So consider that when you begin to look for love.

***The monumental transformation: Adolescence***

Just as we grow and mature from children into adolescents and then into adults, so does our awareness and understanding of love grow and mature. As children, girls typically clump with girls and boys with boys. We learn the ways of friendship in this era, and it seems very important to identify "best friends," to be able to feel we are special enough to rate such and to bond with another human being. So we can see readily that this is all part of our species' make-up, both social and chemical.

And that is one reason that it has become so tragic that activities that used to be important tools for boys and girls to learn good social behavior in general and good interaction skills in close proximity to one another, such as ballroom dancing lessons, have, in the main, been abandoned. For instance, though despised by one and all because it broke the known model of behavior, activities like learning to dance used to begin the bridging of the gap between the distaste children typically feel for those strange creatures of the other sex and the realization that there might, indeed, be a "positive" in the very nature of that difference. These days, in large part, boys and girls simply remain apart and a mystery to one another.

Sure, there are "new" things that have come along, such as girls playing on boys baseball teams and other such "equal" activities, but are these aimed at teaching lessons in interaction between the sexes or are they still functioning as an assertion of equality, not yet having matured into something more productive for the long-term?

It is my belief that this "hole" in our current education for children and adolescents actually aggravates the social situation as children enter adolescence and hormones begin to pump into action. The reaction to the sudden appearance of "forbidden fruit" – driven by our "pornographic" advertising, with the advocacy of casual sex as something considered "normal" by most communications media – without any training in social etiquette, i.e. knowledge of restraint mechanisms – causes many young people to rev up their sexual engines into high gear, and away they go, long before they're prepared to handle such relationships.

This stage, as any parent knows, is also utterly critical in a young person's development. And the capability of parents to help their children through this development crisis ranges all over the place. Some parents layer guilt so completely over an adolescent's emerging sexuality that the child never recovers. Some – many – parents simply leave children to fend for themselves as they ride their hormonal roller coaster and "hope" for the best. Many argue violently with their children over evolving events, causing the family structure to crack and strain.

All the terror and suspense and anger, of course, is over sex – what consequences might occur if a son or daughter becomes sexually active or "what people might say," etc.

Virtually no one during this period talks about love.

That's actually a falsehood. There is endless talk about love – certainly on the part of teenagers, young women especially, who are caught in a social whirl measured by stern evaluation by their peers – Do they have a boyfriend? Are they going steady? Are they popular? Are they going to die of "zits"? And what will that do to their chances of getting a boyfriend? The romantic nature of young women at this age is actually quite endearing – give or take their harsh judgment of/by their peers.

On the boys' part, they, of course, are playing their own peer pressure games, all focused around their shocked amazement at the transformation of their penis and the capabilities it has now gained. Their attention has become rather focused, and they have very little in the way of gradations in emotion about the difference between love and sex. If asked to describe the difference, the universal teenage boy answer would typically be something obtuse like "Yes!" – probably with a fair amount of panting thrown in.

Adolescence truly is a crisis and a mega-turning point in human life. The experimentation in relationships, which will build patterns for virtually all the rest of one's life, today unfortuantely happens by accident for the most part. If there is any talk of love and respect and trust, it most likely will come from individuals and institutions that very often appear to teenagers like repressive people who never experienced what they are currently experiencing. They will be seen as offering teenagers sterile and useless advice and counsel that is simply targeted at containing and controlling them "forever," with the "real intent" to make them live empty and miserable lives, exactly at a time when their bodies are shouting Walt Whitman's refrain, "I sing the body electric!"

To a teenager, that is not very welcome advice.

Sadly, at just the point when adolescents could use solid knowledge about the nature of love and how sex plays a role in that, most – at least from what I have observed in life – go without, and while there will be those who figure it out on their own, there will be those who don't and who will go down the years of their lives never knowing there's a difference between sex and love and who will miss completely what love could mean in their lives. The real sadness is that we as a society think betraying our children through such irresponsibility is "normal." We feel the crude "boot camp" analogy – it happened that way to me, so you should have to suffer the same – is reasonable in dealing with what is probably some of the most important education we should provide.

What teenagers ought to know is that their bodies and minds are beginning to change to prepare for something even far more remarkable than they're experiencing now, as amazing and astonishing as the feelings might be. And the ups and downs of the mood swings of adolescence is, in fact, one's mind and body coming into a new synchronization that will eventually even out to yield wonderful results a teen can't yet imagine, if he or she will let the development happen fully.

A good analogy to use might be that of a fireworks rocket that's about to take off. When first lit, many fireworks give off some wonderful and beautiful sparks as the chemicals and heat come to life. But are these first sparks – as amazing as they might seem – anything to compare to the moment the rocket blazes across the sky in its glory? Should one really squander one's excitement and joy at a few sparks rather than letting the whole wonderful change occur to oneself and then riding that rocket to the emotional heights that are the real reward of love?

Many teens will have a hard time believing that something better is on its way because of the power of what they are experiencing, and will simply squander their growth and development, and many are the class reunions where people recognize the classmates who "bloomed early" and wasted their potential. These individuals never really got past the sexual changes to their body and settled for an empty repetition of a physical act that – while wonderful – never takes them to the moon, as they would easily travel if they'd learn the ways of love at least as well as they'd learned the ways of sex.

The adolescent phase, and the seemingly endless process of falling in and out of "love" as one's emotions surge, if understood correctly, can be seen as a time providing terrific "practice" for the day one eventually collides with real love, for one has been learning through this process to "let go" emotionally, bit by bit, an essential process for actually falling in love.

***Young adulthood – the real time to start looking for love***

By the time one has reached one's twenties, the chemical/biological transformation of the human body is complete. But what has it really achieved? Two things:

- First, we are physically complete in being able to carry on the species, and, emotionally – while still having a lot of immature elements to grow out of through experience – we are stable enough to begin raising children, if we so desire. (A lot of society's problems could be resolved easily if people would have children *because they desire them* rather than because their parents want grandchildren, or society expects it of people to be "normal," i.e. ever notice what a menacing and guilt-inducing question "Do you have any children?" is?)

- Second, and more important for the pursuit of love, one's body has created an amazing "detection" system that is constantly analyzing data received from other people – physical form, "glances," smells, etc. – and interpreting that data as to the potential a person represents as a mate. This data is also compared to an "ideal" form one has been developing deep in the mind throughout one's life from many influences, and consists of what that ideal person looks like, acts like, etc.

People who fall in love at first sight and who simply "know" they've connected with the right person are more than likely seeing an imposition of their mental ideal fitting almost perfectly with a living human being. When such happens, two people come into perfect synchronization immediately and that's all there is to it. It does happen.

But for most of us that isn't going to happen. The person we come to love may have many of the attributes we have configured as part of our ideal, but he or she doesn't match quite perfectly. The good news is that it doesn't really matter. The template we develop is just that, a model to help us sort through the mass of humanity in searching for someone that we know we could love, and if we've lined up a fair number of those attributes, that's sufficient for finding a good mate.

This may sound a little offbeat, but as a way to understand how our minds are working in trying to help us get to love, think of becoming an adult as the same as human beings blossoming like a flower with hundreds, if not thousands, of little antennas blossoming out of our heads. As we move through the world, these sensitive instruments are endlessly looking to match up with similar antennas on other humans.

As they test the waters, first by simply seeing people, then during the process of dating, without even having to trouble yourself much about it, these antennas go about seeing how many matches they can find. They do this by "touching" the antenna on the other person. When enough nerve points are hit, when a sufficient number have achieved "desirability" – Wham-O! – the phenomenon of love begins to take place. Your brain's data analysis system begins saying to you, "Hey! There's a critical mass here, enough emotional points to create love, so it's being unleashed."

And, suddenly, when that happens, you begin a journey into a world you previously had no way of knowing existed. One begins the process of "falling" towards the person who has set off your "love alarm" system: You think about them almost every minute of the day. You can't bear to be apart from them. You spend time that should be used for other things writing notes to them, or figuring out some strategy to please them so they'll love you even more.

Your life becomes consumed by the other person, and you keep "falling," getting closer and closer and more intimate in your conversations and ways of behaving. Interest in what other people are doing – unless it's arranging some event that can be another excuse for the two of you to get together – becomes less and less meaningful. Even your best friends don't mean quite the same to you as they once did.

What your "love system" that you were given during the change in adolescence is doing is, in fact, operating to make you fall towards the one you love. Think of those antennas touching and winding around one another. The more antennas that touch and intertwine and pull together, the stronger the pull gets, just as one strand of hair is really nothing, but a handful being pulled all together has a great deal of strength and solidity to it.

And that's the job of these emotional antennas. If enough of them connect and pull two people together tightly, the two will bond and fuse into one entity and, ideally, stay together for always. And that's what you hope for in love. You're looking for that puzzle piece that's been missing from you since you came into adolescence – and which has caused that constant ache from lack of love. And when you bond thoroughly in love, that void, that ache, does go away.

What's even more wonderful is that it gets replaced, only this time with a contentment and a serenity and a happiness that you can't even imagine existed before you found – that's right – love. Only by getting to love can you know this feeling. But you have to have the courage to let go and let the process happen naturally to get to love.

***Failing at love without even meaning to…***

People are, of course, naturally afraid that if they let go emotionally, they might be hurt, because one makes oneself vulnerable in the process. That's why I recommend wholeheartedly learning to love first before rushing off to a bedroom or the back seat of a car. At the risk of sounding like one of those uptight people trying to force control on young people, I can only observe that one is far less likely to find oneself feeling used and possibly abused by ending a relationship that is not working before sex than afterwards. The all-too-common belief that fundamental problems will somehow "disappear" or be "worked out" by having great sex typically brings only ruin upon a relationship when the issues should have been worked out in advance or people should have moved on.

Plus, in an age where the sexes have been virtually pitted against one another as something "normal," thanks to our popular culture, many cannot get across this important bridge to trust and opening up to another person because they cannot deal with the apparent paradoxes of love. For instance, many of us have been turned into "control freaks" by modern life. Not only do we not like to "lose control" but the relationship between men and women has been turned into something viewed as a struggle for control – a battle over who has power in a relationship.

And, in playing such games, one of the most stunning developments in this area is that many people now take the view that the faster he or she can "reject" someone, the "stronger" they are, which, of course, leads one quickly to the conclusion that "all the good men have been taken or are gay" or "all women are bitches." And where, exactly, do people who engage in such a practice think they'll end up in terms of possessing a relationship? This phenomenon is particularly common among those belonging to matchmaking organizations, where, because of their previous negative experiences, tend to view the latest match as merely a piece of "meat" to judge and, more than likely, discard, since "there's more where they came from," which merely reinforces their negative belief system. For it is a fact of life that if one is always looking for the worst in a human being rather than the best, one may be sure one will always find what one is looking for.

In the case of love, the greatest paradox is that the only way to conquer is to yield, to let go and flow into the other person's very being. But who can permit themselves to do this in our time? Our newspapers, magazines, TV, films, and books all tell us that we're surrounded by "stalkers" and others planning to murder or do other vile things to us. And if one or the other person – or both – won't let go and yield, then love will simply never happen.

Sometimes in these circumstances love – in a very flawed form – can exist. A great example of this is the love between musical genius Hank Williams, Sr., and his wife Audrey. Their love was even monumental love – Hank's songs prove it. But the painful misery in being so completely out of balance as their love was created a roller-coaster ride of ecstasy and agony on the part of the two.

One can readily imagine the kind of gigantic and happy love that would have existed if Hank and Audrey had been able to get themselves "in sync." But the irony is that if that had happened, we would not have the extraordinary music – the poetry in Hank Williams' lyrics often stands right next to William Shakespeare's sonnets in the depth of emotion captured – that was created as a result of that flawed love, as Hank Williams tried to deal with his anguish.

But think about it – is that what you want? Love turned into nightmare? If you and the one you're interested in will take the time to get to know each other's essential person first and learn to truly trust one another, then, when love hits, you'll both find it very easy to ride with it. You'll have no problem "letting go" completely and taking your journey to real love.

This seems such a simple and reasonable approach to take, but with all the societal pressures now saying, "Sex first, worry about love – if it even exists – later," it becomes very hard for people to have the courage to wait for love to arrive before letting go emotionally. And that, sadly, is the same thing as saying "bye-bye" to love in the majority of instances before one even arrives at that much-sought-after destination. You'll fall "in sex" instead of "in love."

People who fall in love as the first phase of their relationship know when it's time to express their feelings through sex, which is what sex should be about. Sex then becomes far more powerful and magical than a quick roll in the hay, which is about all you'll ever get from the former method.

# 7. WHAT DOES IT FEEL LIKE TO BE IN LOVE?

♥ This is the part you've been waiting for... This chapter is the central point of this book. Indeed, it's the whole point.

So let me tell you what you're longing to know.

First, the reason love has been so hard to describe throughout history is that its realization so short-circuits the mind that people are usually too swept away to be able to describe it. Plus, since so much of love consists of feelings that seem inarticulate, there is a lot of dancing around the subject as a way to at least "sort of" capture the experience. And, lastly, when love arrives, most people come to the rather profound conclusion that their love is unlike any other love that has ever existed and is unique to the two lovers, which is something at least partially true.

***What it feels like to be in love***

So what is it? What is love? Be prepared to be shocked: It's a doorway into a parallel universe that is identical to this one and superimposed right on top of the world you've always known. You know you've passed through the door because the dull ache that people feel virtually every day of their lives from loneliness is gone. You know you're there because even on the darkest days, colors are brighter; your spirit is lighter; there's an upbeat and positive mood that did not exist before.

You also know it because you can see back into that old world and can observe the loneliness and sorrow of most lives and you're sad to see that people either do not have – or may never have – the extraordinary feeling you possess.

The change is absolutely fundamental to your being. And the conclusion you reach is that such a state is the most natural and wonderful in the world. Why would anyone *not* want to be in love? And to those who were so afraid love would be claustrophobic, it comes as the most wonderful surprise that you have suddenly been liberated – liberated from the pain of ordinary life, liberated to pursue your dreams with solid support behind you, liberated to relish every moment of being alive, for you have someone to share it all with, and life is not some chore or burden that needs to be "managed" to minimize the pain.

Your house or apartment takes on a whole new feel with another life in it – somehow it no longer is a collection of "things," but an environment which has warmth and a living presence about it.

It's truly astonishing that so many don't understand the power that resides in having someone to do something for…to strive and to achieve for – not selfishly for yourself alone, but as a testament to another human's devotion.

In short, another human being in your life gives purpose and meaning to life.

In another of love's paradoxes, by "letting go" and letting your life join with another person's, one (meaning two-in-one) has gained more control over life than they ever imagined possible as separate individuals. Suddenly, there is a calm center to everything – the noisy chaos outside seems foolish and pathetic as people scurry aimlessly about seeking fulfillment in things that will never really bring it. Your entire vision of the world makes a huge shift. You can see in a way you didn't know existed.

Having achieved this through love, now try and imagine what sex becomes to two people using it to express their love for one another as they function on this new level of existence and communication.

***Past the beginning***

What you've been hearing are all aspects of the *beginning* of love. So if that's true, what comes next?

If you take the point of view that you've embarked on an ever-changing journey that is powerful enough to last a lifetime, you'll be prepared to reap the riches that are to come. And if you recognize that so much of what love is about is communication between two lovers, then you'll realize the tools you have to work with – words, sex, acts of kindness, listening, comforting, encouragement, thoughtful gifts, etc. – are all means to foster the growth of your love.

Things you might have thought would be incidental become enormously important – like sleeping together all night, as you realize that doing such is reassurance that someone loves you so much that they will fly through the night with you and be there for you in the morning. Suddenly, that simple act carries a weight of importance right up there with sex itself.

And a lot of the changes that occur with love have to do with vision. If you will imagine the beginning of love as two people starting a journey up a mountain, always climbing upwards towards the top together, you soon come to realize that your view of the world gets better and better and better as you go. It takes very little time at all to begin to understand the emotional heights to which one can climb.

A good way of understanding just how powerful these emotions can grow to be over time is to look at an example – with a superb one being the opera "Carmen." This opera is the story of a beautiful woman – Carmen – who works in a cigarette factory. Carmen has "been around" and thinks she's pretty sophisticated about men and the ways of the world, being quite the manipulator of men. When Carmen's life collides with an ordinary soldier and the impact of their lives catapults the two skyward to monumental love, without any of the growth stages in between, at first Carmen is delighted and staggered by the intensely powerful emotions of such a love. But as time passes, she becomes frightened by emotions of such magnitude and feels so out of control with her life that Carmen comes to the conclusion that she'd rather die than deal with such deep feelings.

The emotions one can achieve – and which can usually only be reached by growing through time together – are extraordinary. And the view of the world one achieves as well confirms the glory of knowing such a love. And this wonder of love unfolds itself like a flower over time, providing continual delight. And the real wonder is that love *does* just keep getting better. While the discovery of love seems enough of a gift itself, with nothing more ever seeming to be needed, it really doesn't happen that way, and love just keeps maturing into something better – and different – with each passing year.

And so, as we grow up through the years into our 30's, 40's, 50's and beyond, love grows with us, regardless of what point in our life we start. It is always new. It is always different. And it will always be something else tomorrow and the day after that. Could anyone get much luckier than that? If we are wise, when we get to love, we will do whatever must be done to nurture it and make love grow and blossom.

***The measure of monumental love***

Hard as it may be to imagine, since any impact with true love seems beyond imagining, love has the capacity to function at a truly monumental level. We tend to call these loves "great love affairs" and remember them as clearly being unusual – Anthony and Cleopatra; Abelard and Heloise; Elizabeth and Robert Browning; and, in fiction, Romeo and Juliet; Scarlet O'Hara and Rhett Butler; and on and on. There is something special about being able to function at such a level.

Monumental love is, in fact, something of a rare flower, like an orchid blooming in a garden of glorious roses. But it is not really different in kind, merely in degree. Its existence in no way takes away from the value and power of love as most people experience it. Monumental love is more about the fact that there are certain kinds of personalities that can deal with emotions of a depth and range that might make others uncomfortable – and whose love is able to grow and develop at a more rapid pace and arrives fairly rapidly at such a height.

Monumental love – since all love is part of a continuum – is also what every love is climbing upwards towards as the years go by. What's really far more important to lovers is to grow their love at their own pace, at a speed that continues the happiness they first found in discovering love. As one sees in the example of "Carmen," rushing into deep waters buys no one much good. But it's worth knowing that monumental love does, indeed, exist, for it serves as a goal, as an aspiration.

And while few will admit to it, monumental love is also a form of love that is highly visible to others. Monumental love is typically marked by a serenity and assurance that most can't quite fathom exists. Such lovers are very self-contained, and their view of life is equivalent to sitting atop Mount Everest where they serenely contemplate the world, living life according to their terms, which simply are the terms that bring them happiness. All the wants and desires fostered by our culture become meaningless measures, and even the thought of desiring another human outside that love appears completely ridiculous and as foolish a concept as could ever be conceived.

Unfortunately, a common reaction to monumental love by average people is that – at least from an outsider's point of view – this extraordinary state is ***so*** desirable when recognized that people will rationalize it is reasonable to do extremely foolish things to try and capture one of the parties in that love, thinking that if they could just get so-and-so, then they, too, could know such astonishing feelings as they are witnessing first-hand.

It never crosses these people's minds that when two people feel so completely whole and complete as one loving entity, any interest in finding someone else is the very last thing to cross their minds. But, typically, many who try to "crash" a monumental love believe it could be "so much better" with him or her in it, so they will try nevertheless. In one sense, one can't blame such people. They know they'll probably never see such a love again, just as they have probably never seen such a love before. So why wouldn't it be worth taking the risk to try and get to it?

But these people are generally the very same people not willing to do what it takes to get to love in the first place, so they never conceive that they'd be doomed to failure were they to succeed.

### ***All love lifts one up***

Monumental love is – for all of us – most important as a demonstration of how tight the bonds can grow from the moment when two people first "let go" to fall in love and how high one can reach in emotional satisfaction. The bond between humans who have found true love simply grows tighter and tighter over the years. And as that spiritual bond pulls them closer, lovers go higher and higher up the emotional curve, carrying them to ever-new and ever-higher levels of emotional satisfaction, and on into a wondrous world that those who never fall in love cannot even begin to realize exists.

## THE LEVEL OF EMOTION THAT CAN BE ACHIEVED FROM VARIOUS LIFE CHOICES

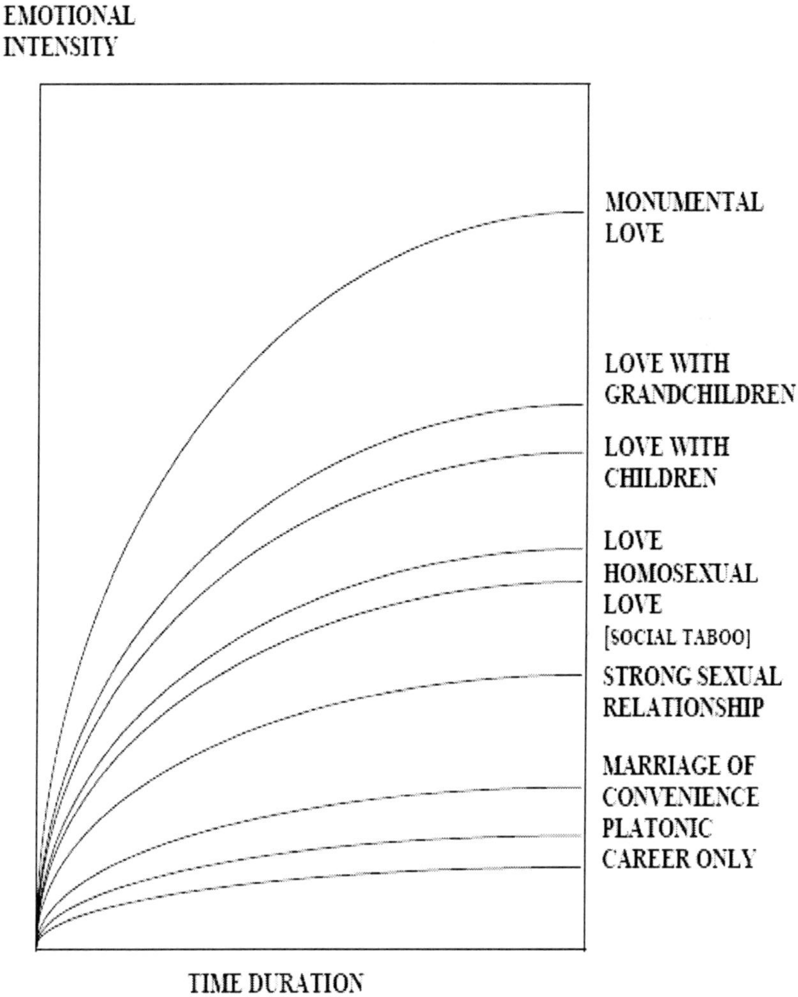

This, then, is what love is. And those who have been there cannot even begin to imagine living without it.

So, now that you know, do you *really* want to believe – as every TV show, as every book, as every magazine says – that love doesn't exist? Are the "smart" people the cynics who deny love really exists or the ones who live their lives in that parallel universe of happiness and contentment known as love?

# 8. SEX – WHERE EXACTLY DOES IT FIT IN?

♥ Many people reading this book may wonder, I'm sure, why this wasn't the first chapter. Or you perhaps turned to this chapter right away. After all, that's the exciting part of love, isn't it? Just the word "sex" itself is titillating. What might this author say that would stir the imagination and give a thrill?

Sex is thrilling, there's certainly no doubt about that. From the first stirring of awareness when one is a juvenile to old age, the subject will be discussed ad infinitum. And one is aware of sex all day through as one observes other people – are they pretty or handsome? How are they responding to me? Look at the way she's looking at him! Etc.

The difficulty of discussing sex is that the subject connects with our animal nature, with our deepest instincts towards keeping the species going. It's virtually impossible to talk objectively about it. A truly objective conversation about sex usually kills the sexiness of sex, turning the discussion into the equivalent of a medical clinic exam that's boring as all get out. If the discussion keeps the "sexiness" to it, the stimulation makes the situation awkward.

The net result is that while the talk in our lives goes on and on about sex, not much is really said or accomplished. There's a popular myth that those who are talking really aren't getting any, and those who aren't talking are busy doing.

There's certainly no doubt that there are those men and women who are skilled at getting others into bed with them. And they are viewed – at least the men, the double standard for women hasn't entirely died – as "heroes." And it is wonderful for most of us to imagine what it would be like to get all the sex we'd like to have. After all, it's so…so…thrilling. And it is – to a point.

What many discover who pursue – and get – all the sex they want for the sake of the physical pleasure it evokes, often find over time that the novelty of sex can wear off. Without the lure of romance – ever notice that people are often more erotic with clothing on than without? – the act of sex becomes just that – an act. Repeating it over and over and over has some benefit, but one's sense of stimulation will become dulled after a great deal of repetition and it just won't seem to be as much fun any more.

Those who continue on such a course soon find they are doing more extreme sorts of things to "get the thrill back." Some even engage in painful acts – and the farther they go, the more they need to add severity to keep things sexually exciting. Most who follow such a path like to view themselves as sophisticated, but the real word that fits the largest majority of such circumstances is, sadly, "jaded."

It is particularly hard for a young person just becoming aware of the astonishing reality of sex to believe that something so monumental and transforming in nature could ever become boring and routine. Sex is one of God's great gifts to Humankind, they think, how could such ever be anything but the most exciting thing in the world? Well, it can.

In fact, for much of the world today, thanks to contemporary advertising, movies, music, television, novels, etc., we've actually headed down the road en mass towards empty sex as a "solution." With so many doubting the reality of love, and stating such as a "fact," it's been concluded that the obvious answer to human needs is to pursue casual sexual coupling as a "normal" means for "releasing sexual tension."

Cruel as it may sound – and many will condemn me for saying this, for they will view it as criticism of their lifestyle – the typical expression of sex today whereby two people grunt and groan like a couple of animals and then walk away to do it again with others when "they need sexual release" is, quite exactly, what most animals do.

In short, the dead-end that sex can become for humans if they pursue sex as their sole goal is merely the reduction of oneself to one's basic animal nature, and is not some "superior" level of sophistication, as many would like to believe. Most people don't like to consider humans as animals, but we are – regardless of our level of development – a living, breathing organism like any other. And many other species enjoy sex as well. It's all a part of the endless chain of life maintaining itself. And maybe to a large number of people, that's all they need in this life. I'm just suggesting there's more if someone wants it.

That's because humans have another part of us that at least appears unique to our species. And that is the fact that we have a spiritual component to us, which is the part of our being that can carry us to love.

Upon hearing that, at this point I'm sure there are quite a few readers ready to bail out, for those words may sound suspiciously like moving to an uptight preacher's harangue on the "law of the missionary position" and a syrupy morality lecture that hasn't got a thing to do with sexy sex.

Wrong. Keep reading. For this is exactly where it gets good.

As mentioned before, the glue of love is communication. And if you will go talk to any human or animal behaviorist, he or she will be more than happy to tell you that sex is a form of communication. And people in love – real love – are doing far more than grunting like a couple of pigs when they are engaging in sex and "releasing their sexual tension."

When sex is so charged with intense emotions, it's really hard to imagine any kind of gradations in that intensity. "It is what it is," many will say. But it's not…

People in love are communicating their "oneness" to each other. They are seeing the depths of the universe in each other's eyes. They know how to let go to feel their emotions to the very depths of their souls. They are engaging in what is probably the most profound religious act on this planet and are at a mental altitude that can easily make them feel this is the closest possibility that exists to knowing God.

You must consider that on a day-to-day basis, as has already been observed, people in love are already walking around in the stratosphere looking down upon those poor mortals who haven't the least idea of how to get up and fly. While those with feet of clay are living out their lives scrabbling about the Earth in their misery, lovers are flying through life. If there's that much of a mental distinction in ordinary human activities, try and imagine what occurs when real lovers know the time is right to grab one another and to fly to the stars.

And, if you doubt what I say, do you really think people are typically going to run around telling others about what they're experiencing? But rest assured, it is an amazing feeling to look out on the world and to know what you know.

Now, for the "pragmatists" among us who will point fingers at what they believe is a hopeless romantic, there is a phenomenon that will occur over time – never forget that love is always evolving, it is never static – about which people should be aware. The most passionate and frequent lovemaking typically occurs within about the first two years of a relationship.

Everything is new. Everything is exciting as two people get to know and love and bond with one another. Then, as things get a bit more routine, there's just not the same urgency to have sex. It's not that it's not fun, or no longer enriching, or anything else of the sort. It's just that the sense of desperately needing to get to love is replaced with a sense of assurance that one's love will always be there.

Think of it this way: Do you really believe you could sustain the intense emotions of the Christmas holidays all the year long? That kind of intensity becomes wearing on one after a while, as much fun as Christmas – or whatever holidays you celebrate – can be. The shift that occurs in one's sexual interest and needs makes a change from being a long-term emotional blast of Christmas to being the special treat of a Valentine's Day. In other words, one no longer feels quite the need to gorge on the Christmas feast, but finds a romantic Valentine Day's treat of candy something very special, indeed.

It does not mean one is no longer in love, or that one loves any less. It is that the shape and dimension of love changes and becomes something new, and that is true as a couple grows together over the years.

An interesting parallel to note is that a large number of marriages – most, in fact, today – can't make it past the two-year mark. People become disillusioned with the change occurring in one another, feeling rejected, undesirable, or a lot of other negative emotions. The change is not viewed as part of the natural evolution that loves goes through, thereby setting things up for disappointment and disillusionment. How could they even know this is part of a natural pattern, when no one has ever drawn for them the model of how love grows and develops?

What this disillusionment can also, unfortunately, mean is that a couple did not fall in love in the first place, but fell "in sex," instead. People whose chief interest is not the person he or she married, but the wonderful romp in bed they achieved with that person, pretty much is on a track to disillusionment anyway, whether it's two years down the road or twenty.

The common error in belief that physical intimacy is the same as real intimacy – which is true emotional connection, a mental bonding with another human being – has led many astray in the belief that they have found love, when what they really have found is temporary, wonderful sex.

It can be a very rude awakening, in fact, to open one's eyes one morning next to someone who is a complete stranger when you thought – and sincerely believed – that you knew the person lying there beside you extremely well. To many, this sensation comes as a real shock of betrayal, with one easily tending to forget that relationships are a two-way street, and their partner probably feels the same. What a hollow, empty feeling that can be.

But for the lovers, for those who have chosen to truly combine their spirits and to bond into one organism through love, the changes that occur across a lifetime in one's sexual needs and desires are taken in stride, because they understand the shifts have nothing to do with anything except in the manner one is expressing their love. For these people, making love will always remain making love. Sex will remain a *means* to a wonderful end and will never cause problems by being the sole objective, especially when believing the latter can so frequently be the path to disaster.

The "Catch-22" of the whole argument being presented is that the people who know what I'm talking about don't need to be told, and the ones who do need to listen will probably think I'm lying. The only observation that can be made in this situation is that people who are truly in love feel an overwhelming sorrow for those who argue persistently against the case for love. And if you're not willing to work to find love, you'll never get there.

The good news, if one wants to call it that, is that the naysayers can die quite satisfied in the assurance of their outlook, for the only way to know love exists is to get there, to experience it directly. Why people would settle for rhinestones when diamonds are right there for the taking, I don't know. But an awful lot of men and women make just that decision. And an awful lot of people waste an awful lot of energy they might be using to find love in arguing the case against it to justify the behavior patterns they choose to follow.

The ultimate lesson is that sex is a means to an end, and not an end in and of itself, regardless of how nice the tingly feeling may seem. Using sex to express your love – as so many poets have tried to tell us – is taking a ride to paradise. It is not just a means to "release one's sexual tension."

A sage piece of advice to remember – this is the only true preaching you'll hear from this author – is that if one wants to gain the most from one's sexual being, the best solution is to "Make love first, then make sex to express your love."

And if I'm not mistaken, instead of that wisdom being common knowledge, there's really only one part of that phrase that's conveyed to us today by every communications media we possess. Does the expression "make sex" sound familiar?

How different our world might be if people had as their first goal to find love, if humans were to make love a higher priority than sex as the premier human experience. Can you imagine the happiness that would thus be generated by those humans then moving on to sex?

Look around you. Can it really be that so many are willing to settle for so little – and actually think they are “smart” in doing so? You’ve been shown the choices and the impact each choice makes on human lives. Which will YOU choose?

# 9. HOW DO YOU KEEP YOUR LOVE ALIVE?

♥ This is a subject about which an enormous amount has already been written. When one goes through a bookstore, it's almost shocking to see how many volumes are dedicated to just this subject, which indicates how many human relationships must be in desperate need of repair. There sure are an awful lot of "first aid kits for love" out there.

We live in a time that seems to place very unusual pressures on relationships – the expectations alone are hard to deal with. So much of the communications between people and the sexes as a whole often seems entirely "out of sync." With all of the conflicting signals and "advice" as to what's right or wrong that abounds, it can be hard to see the way clearly in order to grow and develop one's love in a healthy and positive manner.

The real goal should not be to fix anything, but to prevent harm from happening to a relationship in the first place. If one is lucky enough to find love, one should want to nurture and help it grow and develop, rather than having to always take action when love runs into rough waters or, worse, goes aground upon the rocks.

So what I offer are a few basic concepts to apply to help avoid ever getting to such a stage of distress, and a handful of ideas that will carry you and your love a long way if you will just apply them.

**♥ Expect that your love will change and evolve over time.**

People who make an assumption that love is "one thing" and will always be exactly the same – static – are setting themselves up for disappointment. As has already been shown, love is a journey and not a destination. If you're traveling the road correctly, it gets stronger and richer and more valuable to you with each passing year. The thrill you experienced as a person in your 20's will not be the same – and would you really want it to be? – as the deeper experience you can achieve in your 30's, 40's, 50's and beyond.

**♥ Money problems have destroyed more love relationships and marriages than anything else. Take proactive action to prevent this from ever becoming your problem.**

One of the reasons that money is so consistently a problem is that, for whatever strange reason, teaching money management to young people – unless one's parents care to do this – is something completely ignored in educational systems in the United States of America, a most peculiar phenomenon for a Capitalist society in which money is paramount. Instead, we offer young people easy credit they don't know how to manage, and the next thing they know, they've begun a life's journey enslaved with a mountain of debt, from which they never escape.

If you know nothing about money – or even if you think you do – make learning financial skills a foremost priority:

1. Get one of the financial computer programs like "Quicken" or something similar, and LEARN HOW TO USE IT TO CONTROL YOUR MONEY!!

2. Take a "Personal Financial Management" course which are conducted by colleges and other groups in their continuing education programs, and have your children get involved with programs like Junior Achievement.

If you learn to manage money, you will have one of the greatest defense mechanisms against harm to your love and marriage that you could ever possess. The weight of financial problems is crushing and never-ending when you have them. You can – and will – be subjected to the most unbelievable psychological harassment when your debts mount – and this will be by the very same people who treated you so kindly in offering you easy credit in the first place. Never assume these people are your friends – they are not – they are a business out to make money – and lots of it – at your expense.

How powerful is personal financial control and management? Let's just say that if you don't pay a bit of attention to anything else I write in this entire book, but do what I suggest in learning how to manage your money, you will have made the best investment in your entire life by buying this book.

**♥ Depend upon one another, and not upon anyone outside your love or marriage.**

While it is sometimes valuable to obtain experienced knowledge or advice and counsel from experts outside your love, never forget that the point of two-becoming-one is to create a world that is yours and yours alone. When you come home and close the door, you should forget what others are doing outside – their judgments, their opinions, their ideas on what's right or wrong – and you and your love should discuss and decide what's best for the two of you and the life you have created.

People who live by the dictate "What will people think?" or "What will people say?" are living their lives for complete strangers – most of whom won't even give a damn about what happens to the two of you – and are making decisions based upon a false premise. Yes, it is wise and important to have a good reputation. Yes, it is wise and good to meet community standards in terms of things like maintaining one's home to a reasonable standard. But to live one's life always trying to impress others or to try and keep up with others – which can often mean spending money one does not really have – drains energy from a love and marriage that would be far better used in advancing the needs and dreams of that love.

When times are bad – and there will be bad times; all people of any rank or station in life will experience misfortune at one time or another – the person to turn to is the one you love. Depending upon one another in times of crisis will deepen – not weaken – the bonds between two people. If you find it easier to run away in times of personal crisis, then the roots of your love don't run very deep in the first place. "Always be there for one another" is a first rule of lasting love.

**♥ The love of your life should also be the best friend in your life.**

This sounds very similar to what I just said. And it is related. But marriage counselors have found time and again that people who have married and lived together for many long years can end up finding themselves to be complete strangers. This is often the case regarding people who have "fallen in sex" rather than fallen in love, who assume – because the erotic side of their life is so intense and enjoyable – that they know one another "intimately," or it can also result from having married from pressure from family or from other societal forces.

Always consider: "What do I have in common with this person I'm attracted to? What do we really have to talk about after a romp in the hay? Do I really like the person inside that body?" That's the person one should be falling in love with.

A human shell is just that – a shell – one that will fade and wither with time. So ask this, too: "When that happens, as it will to all human beings, will I take such happy pleasure in knowing that person that the fading of physical looks will really make no or little difference to me?"

If you can't answer such questions rather reasonably, then you may be sure that the emotions you are really feeling about that person are not love, however wonderful they may be. People who have not learned to distinguish "falling in sex" from "falling in love" are in real danger of pursuing a beautiful or handsome disaster that will come to fruition somewhere down the road.

♥ **"Always be yourself – if you don't have yourself, then you don't have anything."** ***– Cole Porter, Songwriter***

Songwriter Cole Porter, whose beautiful songs about love provide timeless insight into the nature of love, was a very wise man in many ways. The above statement is one of the profoundest things he ever said. Consider it this way: Do you recall how you felt at one time or another when someone conned you out of money or talked you into doing something you really shouldn't be doing? Didn't you feel rather dirty and used after you'd been "taken" in such a manner?

An essential part of love is falling in love with the inner person of the one you desire. And if you trust and let go – as you must to get to true love – and let yourself fall, don't you think it might be quite a shock to discover the person you are falling in love with isn't really there, and is actually a "false front" put up to disguise the real person?

Also, consider the converse of this: if you feel you have to pretend to be something you're not in order to attract a lover, isn't something sort of wrong with the picture? Wouldn't you do better to make permanent changes to whatever needs fixing rather than pretending? If a person doesn't really like him or herself, why should anyone else?

The dearest possession you will ever have – besides the love of your life – is yourself. One needs to learn to appreciate who and what one is – be proud of your virtues, correct those deficiencies that you can, and understand that everyone has his or her own particular quirks that cannot be changed, but actually help define their personality and will prove very often to be endearing qualities.

If you don't learn to like yourself, it's going to be very difficult to get to love, because you'll always be sitting in judgment of the person who happens to like you. You'll believe they have poor judgment for even choosing you, and then will always doubt their judgment going forward.

And if it turns out someone doesn't happen to like the essential you, then he or she is, quite simply, the wrong person for you anyway, and you're darn lucky to know that. Anyone who approaches love as something less than a lifetime commitment is not really looking for love. And you can't go down an entire lifetime pretending to be something you're not without eventually being caught in the act at some point in time, causing massive disillusionment.

Love, real love, is based upon absolute trust. Being a good actor or actress is not that. Listen to Cole Porter's advice. It's as solid as any you'll ever hear.

**♥ Make sure a man knows you respect him; make sure a woman knows she is loved.**

In the light of the great struggle for human equality that's occurred in our recent history – something I agree with quite completely – there is still, however shocking it may sound to some, a basic difference between the sexes. Duh!

The struggle to reconcile the psychological differences between men and women has actually been going on down through most of history. Whatever the source of the differences – whether it's hormonal or whether it's psychology caused by physical differences – the fact is that men and women have different psychological needs.

Many feminists will argue with the statement I make in the headline about the difference in those needs – indeed, when I presented this argument at a meeting one time, one woman angrily told me that women want to be respected just as much as men. Of course, they do. But I'm still making a valid statement about the differentiation between the sexes in terms of fundamental priorities.

Men's lives revolve around a sense of respect – about their work, about being considered worthy by their girlfriend or wife, about respect from their children, and even their dog. Knowing they possess this respect is far more important to most men than hearing the words, "I love you."

Women, on the other hand, gain a very rich sense of being from the recognition of an intimate awareness of their inner being by the one they love. Hearing the words "I love you" – arguably the most powerful phrase in any language – confirms a purpose and value for their lives to many women.

There is also no question that these are roles and reactions that have been created by thousands of years of history of human behavior and that continue to evolve. What I'm saying is that the priorities for each sex can serve as important guideposts in intimate relationships that can be honored and respected without demeaning either side, and, if honored, will help maintain both the stability and the depth of the love two people experience.

If we make the mistake of addressing these needs in a manner that views them as weakness, or if we refuse to acknowledge and deal with them as one of the "facts of life," or, worst of all, if we choose to turn these principles into a weapon of hurt and control by withholding respect from men or refusing to let women know they are loved, then we are willfully choosing to cripple the progress and development of our love, and, in many cases, to simply kill it because these are absolutely fundamental needs of both men and women.

## ♥ What a Husband Most Needs

"To the female sex: Have you ever wondered what a man most needs from the woman that he loves? Some of you may think it's love; others may say it is companionship. Many of you may say, 'It's got to be sex!' But the fact is, the answer is found in scripture, in God's Word.

"Ephesians Chapter 5, verse 33 says, 'Let each individual among you also love his own wife as himself, and let the wife see to it that she respects her husband.' You see, God has made man and woman with just a little bit of difference in their needs. **The woman most needs love, but the man's greatest need from the woman he loves is respect.** The world beats him down, but you can build him up or tear him down more than anyone.

"I encourage you to remember this. You may find that your man is not only a whole lot happier, but that you receive a whole lot more love in return."

– The Reverend Bryant Wright
*One Minute of Your Time...*
*Right From My Heart*, 1997

## ♥ What a Wife Most Needs

*"Husbands, love your wives, just as Christ also loved the church..."*
*– Ephesians 5:25*

"Dr. James Dobson was asked, 'Why are men so insensitive to women's needs today?' He answered, 'I question whether men have really changed all that much. I doubt if men *ever* responded as women preferred. Did the farmer of a century ago come in from the fields to say, 'Tell me how it went with the kids today?' No. He was as oblivious to his wife's nature then as husbands are today.'

"So men, if you're struggling to meet your wife's needs, the *Bible* gives a few tips:

"**Physical affection.** Not just sex, but a tender touch which may include a few hugs through the day.

"**Security.** Physical, financial and emotional...a wife desires security in all its forms.

"**Understanding.** Listening more than telling her what to do.

"**Reassurance.** Knowing you think she's beautiful, in a society of constant comparison.

"**Spiritual leadership.** Not dictatorship, but servant leadership, like Christ for His church.

"These are what a wife needs most from her husband."

–The Reverend Bryant Wright
*One Minute of Your Time...*
*Right From My Heart*, 2007

**♥ Never, never, never, never, never, never, never go to bed angry at one another.**

In the event you just missed what I just said, it's truly a mistake to go to bed angry with your love, without resolving the problem in some manner. The reason this is so deadly an act is that all through the night the problem will eat away at one's spirit and grow in size. The next morning one discovers there's an even bigger problem than the one you started out with the night before. In the light of dawn, there's more to resolve because one comes to conclude the actions that caused the anger are a betrayal or the harboring of a grudge. A wedge is driven that will grow and grow and grow.

Many people make the serious mistake – though well intended – of concluding that if one "sleeps on a problem" it will be easier to resolve, that it's a calmer, more rational manner of problem solving, rather than blowing up at one another. And that seems logical on the surface. But the essential problem is that you're not dealing with mathematics or a simple matter of logic, you are dealing with human emotions and feelings, which do not necessarily attach themselves to reason, and, in fact, rarely do. Love is a coming together as one, which implies compromise to maintain that single center. Two angry people lying on opposite sides of a bed seething are not "one."

It is best to settle your differences and to apologize to one another for any hurt feelings that have been caused and to go to sleep in each other's arms.

If you cannot fully resolve a problem, a second-best solution is to acknowledge – before going to bed – that a problem has been created, that you will both try to think it through more clearly and offer a compromise solution in the daylight, and that the anger that has been expressed is about the problem and not about the person you love. And most often, that is absolutely true.

However, ***listen carefully:*** When it comes to issues between people, you do have an ***absolute*** guarantee that if you do not come to resolution on a problem, the anger that remains will be about the other person and not about the problem. No manufacturer ever gave a more ironclad guarantee.

Other than learning to manage one's money, no suggestion given within these pages is worth more than what you have just read when it comes to creating a lasting love. You should both be humble enough to remind one another that "We're in this love together, and what do we – as a couple – need to do to solve this problem and put it behind us?"

**♥ Give of yourself – don't give things.**

Many people have a terrible misconception about the nature of giving. They believe that spending money on some sort of gift – any kind of gift – should be more than sufficient to impress another person, and that such is a true demonstration that one cares. But most people – put yourself in this spot – have a really good sense of when a gift comes from the heart, or, sadly, the reverse, when someone in merely "going through forms" in doing their Christmas or Valentine's Day or birthday "duty."

Probably the best articulation of true giving was captured in writer O. Henry's brilliant short story "The Gift of the Magi," which is about a truly loving man and woman suffering hard times, where, unknown to one another, the man sells his beloved pocket watch to buy his wife beautiful combs and brushes she has long admired, and the woman sells her beautiful hair to buy her husband a gold chain for his cherished watch. Each sacrificed their most beloved possession to bring their lover happiness.

Yes, they gave each other material gifts. But the true gift was the spirit behind the giving. That is what people cherish most, not material things, which are mere symbols of a love.

There are people – those with money who can afford to provide lavish gifts often assume this – who have the idea that they really can buy affection through such giving. They can even go to great pains and expense in this kind of giving. But such behavior represents a typical failure in understanding what a gift is all about.

For instance, it can be very easy to develop an expectation where individuals believe they are "owed" love or affection or gratefulness for their gifts, that the point of gift giving is to create some sort of obligation to receive something in return. Unfortunately, while life can work like that in many instances, when it comes to real affection, it does not necessarily hold true.

People who recognize someone is simply trying to buy their attention or affection in this manner – especially if they are made to feel guilty about such gifts by the giver – usually end up offended and resent the giver, interpreting these displays as "showing off" that demonstrates wealth or power and not love. And, quite frankly, such behavior does function as a form of condescension, regardless of how well intended the giver might be, especially if it's the only understanding of "giving" they have known in their life, and they simply don't know better.

Real giving has little to do with money and everything to do with one's spirit and heart. Many is the person who would be more flattered by a homemade card or video testimony of one's love than an expensive jewel. Many is the person who would be happily surprised to walk outside to find a cleanly washed car with a message of love tucked under the windshield than a new toaster.

Giving is placing one's love ahead of oneself in one's thinking. It is considering the loved one as worth doing something special for... It is a belief in thoughtfulness – in taking the time for someone else that might be spent selfishly. It is a testimony of human respect.

If the gift meshes with the loved one's thinking, it is a gift. If it does not, it is merely a material object.

Men, in particular, have a difficult time with giving, because so many do not like to shop – wandering around in stores can seem a very aimless and meaningless exercise. But this dilemma can be easily remedied by listening to one's girlfriend or wife carefully, or one can call their wife's or girlfriend's mother or sister or friend to learn about the kind of gift that might move their love's heart.

Taking the time to do this is as much a demonstration of caring as the gift itself. And giving someone something they'd truly like to have is far better than simply giving an object that will be looked at momentarily and disposed of – regardless of how costly it might be.

There's another side to giving that can mean a lot to many and can generate not only happiness in a relationship, but greater intimacy – little surprises. Think about it. When life swoops down upon you – job, kids, home care, etc. – and the world seems to hem you in, nothing is more wonderful than to simply be remembered.

A note tucked into a pocket or purse; a phone call when it's least expected; a little bouquet of flowers when you've gone to the grocery store to pick up milk – all these types of things are gifts that can mean more than larger gifts at holidays or birthdays, for they are unexpected and break the monotony of life. And, most importantly, they are true gifts from the heart.

This is a form of communication, and thinking about one another, reminding each other of your love, serves admirably to help keep love alive. That is the true purpose of gifts – showing you are thinking about someone, demonstrating your ongoing love to someone, remembering the love that brought you together.

Anything else is just "another toaster." And the failure to understand that, can, in the long run, toast your love.

♥ **Never neglect the power of touch.**

Love – as I have repeated endlessly by this point – is really about communications, some done verbally, some by body language, and some by physical contact – touching. Touching someone is physical confirmation of their reality, of their existence. It is also a means of rebonding. Touching says you like to be with someone, that they are special to you, that their nearness to you is important.

Many people live out their lives rarely touching. They may occupy the same house, but they sail by each other like ships, never coming near, except for an occasional kiss "hello" or "goodbye."

Being "one" together means coming together. It also is good role modeling for when you have children, in order to let them see the importance – and proper role – of touching in a love relationship.

Many people think of touching only in a "dirty" manner – the grabbing of a breast or a buttock, for instance. But that's not what touch is about. Touch is about reassurance, more than anything else.

Consider this: If your husband or wife is sitting reading and you happen to pass by, do you reach out and touch his or her head or shoulder or cheek when you pass by to let them know you notice them? If you happen to be standing together talking, do you ever think to tell your wife or husband, "I could use a hug right now"? If you're riding in a car, do you grab your mate's hand and hold it for a moment or pat them on the leg just to let them know you still care?

Seems like such a little thing, doesn't it? Seems like something people don't think about and often overlook – and that's true. Touching – and, please, this does not mean hanging all over a person – in its best sense, is a habit that can readily be developed and bring deep personal riches in providing knowledge to one another that each is loved. In terms of human psychology, physical touch restores and strengthens repeatedly the bond that has been created between two people when they originally fell in love, something that can dissolve and fall apart from years of living together separately.

**♥ True intimacy is a matter of communications and not just a matter of sex.**

Because of the extraordinarily poor education we receive in the ways of love, it would not be out of line to guess that most people think stripping off all their clothes and diving into a bed together is the most intimate human beings can be. As time can so readily reveal – and has to so many – it's quite amazing to discover that people can do such things and never have the slightest knowledge of one another.

So what is "intimacy?" Intimacy is shared communication at the deepest level possible. It is an open sharing of one's mind with another. The tools we have – honesty, openness, trust, words, behavior, touch, sex – all are a means of reaching intimacy. Clearly, sex can be a deep and profound means of communicating with one's lover, but it is not, in and of itself, an intimate act.

Great loves, which represent a fusing of personalities, a bonding of souls, function on a highly intimate basis, because the two involved are completely "in sync" with each other's thinking and behavior. Signs of this that appear with time and which can be startling to others is just how much is being communicated between two lovers wordlessly, almost as if they can read each other's minds. And, for all practical purposes, they can.

And when such lovers are alone, they can talk in a way that others, who live with each other on a more formal basis, can never achieve. Intimacy, like love, finds its roots in trust. So the net result is that there are probably millions of people who have had sex, had children together, and lived together for years who have never had a second of true intimacy in their lives.

The best analogy I can make is very much like people in a boat off the East Coast of Australia. To the people in the boat, all there seems to be in the world is a big, flat, boring sheet of water that maybe rolls a bit, and that's it. But to the people who wanted more, who trusted to snorkels and aqualungs, and who dove beneath the surface, there's a multi-faceted world of amazing and colorful riches known as the Great Barrier Reef, a thrilling work of nature that is almost beyond description. That is the difference in what people see and experience, if they learn to achieve real intimacy. One MUST go beneath the surface to reach those feelings.

So which world would you prefer to live in and explore? True intimacy – based upon mutual trust between two people – is the doorway to deep emotional riches of love.

**♥ Listen to one another.**

What did I just say? You had to look back at the heading to check, didn't you? Reaching intimacy, maintaining a love is all about communications. Listening is a vital, and I mean vital, part of that process. It is also one of the hardest things in the world for many people to do. What they're usually focused upon is what they're planning to say next.

Merely sitting patiently while someone talks is not listening, however much one might think it is. Listening is a learned skilled. It is also an act of deep caring, in letting someone know that you think they are important. Many are the problems that arise – not because anyone means ill – but simply because someone hasn't been listening when they should.

Couples who sustain a great love for all their life do so because they communicate very strongly and fully in ***both*** directions. They consult one another, weigh alternatives with one another, they are able to deal with issues and concerns with care on both sides.

You will be amazed, if you learn the skill of listening, how much can be learned – and accomplished – by doing just that. But far too many think that listening is a one-way street, and that's a deadly error. Those who talk and expect their mate to listen, but who never have time to listen in return, are asking for grief – and, oddly enough, often end up as people who cannot even begin to understand why they have a problem with their mate.

**♥ The three most powerful words in the world are "I love you."**

If you want to be in love, real love, then it is not an unreasonable expectation to learn how to pronounce those three words and to know when and how to use them.

People NEED to hear those words. I did not say "like" to hear those words, though surely the hearers of that phrase like it. I said people NEED to hear those words.

If you think you're not a writer, and cannot write great letters or poems or any other kinds of expressions of love, fear no more. A note that simply says "I love you" means more than one could say in a million other words. The key is simply to not be afraid to use them.

Fix this in your mind, particularly if you are a man: It is NOT a sign of weakness to say "I love you" to someone. And if you cannot say it, because you do not feel it, or you cannot bring yourself to commit to someone, then you should feel like you're a cad – man or woman – if you persist and use someone in such a manner, always leaving him or her hanging.

Unfortunately, many young men, in particular, will do the very reverse and tell any woman "I love you" if she will just sleep with him, which is just as irresponsible, but hormones are far more important than truth at a young age, and an awful lot of people have been hurt by such lies, so young women should exercise caution.

But the larger problem in our society is that people who cannot use that expression will probably rarely get to love. They perhaps will have mechanical – and sometimes really wonderful – sex. But the failure to comprehend the meaning and power of that phrase, coupled with the fear of commitment – and this is true for both sexes, mind you – will, time and again, have the same effect as building a wall against ever achieving real intimacy and love. You won't get past the front door, much less achieve love, if you can't even admit to love.

**♥ NEVER use guilt or money to control a loved one's behavior.**

Actually, this is a sterling method to kill your love, if you really are foolish enough to want to do that. This behavior is tragically all-too-common practice for many people who believe they will have no control or power otherwise, and that's a mistake. The use of guilt destroys another human's self-esteem, as does holding money over someone's head and are behaviors so serious and destructive that I've often felt that both should be considered crimes.

Just be forewarned – far too many humans use these tools to dictate the behavior of other people. The result will invariably be hatred for the perpetrator, and, if you use this approach, it may well not be long before your former loved one finds respite in someone else's arms. And if you find your love is applying this kind of guilt and/or pressure, have the grit to walk away if you have to, for it is a sure path to bitterness and unhappiness. You have been warned.

**♥ It's the day-to-day grind that can often wound and sometimes kill a love or a marriage.**

To many lovers, love dies when the real world enters into their personal world of love. Love suddenly seems as though it were a transitory fantasy, a wonderful illusion that must – without doubt – be replaced by car payments, baby diapers, and the struggles of work and careers. Today, the matter is complicated by the fact that many couples are now forced to maintain a two-income status if they're to be able to afford a house or lifestyle where they can live with some dignity. As a common effect, the bloom falls off the rose of love and weighty obligation takes its place. That's a simply terrible scenario, but that is, most unfortunately, how life plays out for so many.

Reality – as we all find from time to time – can be quite annoying, since love appears as an ideal state fueled by romantic fantasy that can be difficult to sustain. But if a couple will adapt their perspective to the circumstances, it is possible to turn the day-to-day situation around and to apply love as the "salve" or "balm" to the rigors life imposes upon all of us.

If you view your home life as the shelter from the storm of life – and maintain it on that basis, carefully avoiding letting others dictate to you the "proper" way to live your personal life – and if you will shut out the noise and bother outside your front door when you come home, you can help keep alive a secret world that protects you from the anguish others so willingly want to inflict upon you.

And you can do this in a way that involves your whole family, making each of you important, for children should rightfully be an extension of you and your spouse's love. Children are absolute proof that two can become one.

Here are just a few ideas couples can use to fight back against the day-to-day grind that can wear them down:

- Go on a date with each other regularly. Trying to budget too tightly and ending up always at home can become a habit you may never be able to break. Before, and even after you have children, take time once a month – or at least every quarter – to do something together – alone – if you can. Try and make the event something new and different, so you keep variety in your life.

- Plan an outing that your spouse or love knows you'd hate to do (ballet/fishing), but you know would be very special to your mate. It will help to promote common understanding.

- Remind yourselves of the love that brought you together. If other loves are worth documenting in books, movies, and music, then record yours in words or on video or audio or in a scrapbook as a keepsake for yourselves and as something for your children as a remembrance of their roots and the importance you place on love.

- Realize a dream that each of you has – rather than letting it become something you regret and wish you had done after your mate has died. For instance, if one of you has a dream of seeing Paris, then plan and budget for it and DO it. Give yourselves memories worth having. Memories are, after all, all you'll ever take with you in the end. Collect them.

- Make sure your wife or husband knows you miss them during the day, and that they're the first person you want to see when you get home at night.

- Sleep in the same bed. Unless there is a physical problem that would prevent it, don't make the mistake of not learning to sleep with one another and flying through the night in each other's arms. Many people come to realize that eight hours of such togetherness and reassurance can be worth just as much as – if not more than – sex. To sleep separately is to start heading into separate lives.

- Look in your lover's eyes when you talk. Nothing is so disconcerting as people who cannot look another human being in the face. The eyes are the doorway to the soul. Connect. Communicate in every way you can with the one you love. Don't build uncertainty and fear through avoidance of another's eyes – especially the person you love.

- Have enough respect for yourself and your mate to stay in shape. This does not mean you have to be a bodybuilder. It means having a reasonable appearance that would be attractive to the other sex – and something that will bring happy sex to you as a result.

- Turn off the TV set at least once a week. Nothing turns love into a world of individuals living separately more than television. Spend at least once a week with your loved one. Play cards or board games. Make cookies or pizza together for the kids while they do their homework. Read together. Do ANYTHING but watch TV. What you may find will happen is that you'll come to detest television and its assault of commercials – did you know there are 26 minutes of commercials in every hour? – and you will find better things to do with your time and your family's time. And there are plenty of better things to do.

- Never buy an appliance for a birthday gift. NEVER. Enough said.

- Fill your home with beauty – color and light create a happy and optimistic atmosphere; slovenliness, darkness, and decay give a continual feeling of insecurity and chaos.

- Frame and make a wall of your children's art and change it year by year. Your children are a direct reflection of your love. Make them a part of your love affair.

- Call when you're away from home. If you love someone, can't you take a moment to check on him or her?

- Buy a bouquet of flowers at the grocery store on the way home each Friday to make your home special for the weekend.

- Make a collection of your favorite romantic songs for Valentine's Day for your mate to listen to in the car as a reminder of your love.

- And should temptation ever come your way, be wise and apply the advice of actor Paul Newman, who said, "Why do I want hamburger out when I've got steak at home?"

Get the hint? Be thoughtful. Think of other people – think of your love instead of yourself for a change.

Thinking about the person you love should fill your heart with joy. It should also make you realize how fortunate you are to have such an anchor in the rough times of human life. If you are standing on the foundation of a solid love, then you will have added strength and confidence in facing the challenges in whatever line of work you do when you walk out the door each morning.

***A Last Thought***

The moment one feels the stress on his or her love or marriage has become such that other people and circumstances outside one's relationship are beginning to look better than what one has, that is the moment he or she should realize they've forgotten all about the love that brought two together and they need to take immediate action to protect their love. And if such action is needed, then it may well be time to find professional help or to head to a bookstore to search through the miles of "save your marriage or love" books to find a remedy that may or may not exist. Taking care of one's love is always easier (and more fun) than trying to salvage it.

# 10. WHAT ABOUT HOMOSEXUAL LOVE?

♥ Can homosexuals know true love/monumental love? To many, the answer to this question may come as a shock, and to some it may be offensive, but the answer is a rather blunt "Yes."

The greatest love poems ever written – William Shakespeare's sonnets, poems so powerful one can feel what it was like to be within his love – were written by Shakespeare to another man. The greatest funeral ever held was Alexander the Great's farewell to his soul mate Hephaistion.

The Roman Emperor Hadrian made his lover Antinous into a god, whom many people – of both genders – across the Classical World worshipped. And even in modern times, the extraordinary exploits of Lawrence of Arabia were inspired by and dedicated to his love – an Arab Bedouin.

And though similar love on the part of women has not been documented anywhere as well, the famous love poetry of Sappho is some of the most beautiful in history.

Love, great love, goes beyond the bounds of one's human physical nature and reaches an emotional state that surpasses one's gender.

And while that may all be true, there's still a catch. For example, even the man many would argue is perhaps the greatest mind ever to appear on this planet – William Shakespeare – collided with the social structures, institutions, and beliefs of his time and could not overcome them to maintain his love.

The difficulties of sustaining a homosexual love in our own time – despite all the advances made thus far by the gay liberation movement – is still a road very few travel with success. And the sacrifices one must make – often resulting in the loss of one's family and friends; damage to one's career; limitations on where one might choose to live, etc., which still occur despite the laws that have been passed – often prove very destructive to long-term relationships.

Though things are changing as the concepts of fidelity and marriage are taking hold within the gay community, the traditional pattern of gay culture often still remains the culprit in the ruin of many personal relationships. For example, in the case of men, gay culture – simply in the way it has developed – maintains an overwhelming emphasis on physical appeal and youth. It emphasizes eroticism as strength and love as weakness. It is a culture built around bar-life and late-night hours, which once was the only time gay people could see one another with minimal fear. And there remains an almost "taken-for-granted" expectation that most relationships are going to be short-term, lasting about as long as immediate and intense sexual interest lasts.

There are very definite – and often quite practical – reasons that gay society evolved the kind of culture that it did. And many of these reasons remain quite valid in our social state of development, where many people today still engage in prejudice based upon sexual preference, race, color, or religion as commonplace behavior.

However, the "practical" response by gay culture to prejudice through the behavior patterns that have developed does

TO THE ONLY BEGETTER OF
THESE ENSURING SONNETS
MR. W. H. ALL HAPPINESS
AND THAT ETERNITY
PROMISED
BY
OUR EVER-LIVING POET
WISHETH
THE WELL-WISHING
ADVENTURER IN
SETTING FORTH

***

Sonnet 29

When, in disgrace with Fortune and men's eyes,
I all alone beweep my outcast state,
And trouble deaf heaven with my bootless cries,
And look upon myself and curse my fate,
Wishing me like to one more rich in hope,
Featured like him, like him with friends possessed,
Desiring this man's art, and that man's scope,
With what I most enjoy, contented least;
Yet in these thoughts myself almost despising,
Haply I think on thee, and then my state,
Like to the lark at break of day arising
From sullen earth, sings hymns at heaven's gate;
　　For thy sweet love rememb'red such wealth brings
　　That then I scorn to change my state with kings.

WILLIAM SHAKESPEARE
*The Sonnets*

not lessen the fact that the social structures that have arisen within gay society continue, unfortunately, to leave many men – as they age and their looks fade in a physically obsessed culture – all alone, with a high degree of alcoholism present, and often great emptiness in an individual's personal life because many within gay culture still view love as weakness, and pair bonding as something for those "who can't play the game."

And while I have no real authority to speak concerning Lesbian culture, my observation is that many Lesbian relationships are probably far more successful inasmuch as they can exist in a much more quiet and accepted fashion, and women tend to have a greater sense of the importance and need for companionship than men – as well as being able to establish relationships based upon a romantic tenderness, if you will, which, as I observed, is often viewed as weakness on the part of men.

For the most part – and, again, this is mere anecdotal observation and not scientific fact – it appears to me that most Lesbian relationships are relatively invisible for the most part in comparison to the far more aggressive and vocal male sexual culture (though year by year, the Lesbian movement is becoming stronger, and clearly more visible, as demonstrated by the many Lesbian couples who have come forth as gay marriage has been legalized).

The enormous growth in the homosexual population in our time has been argued in many ways. Many believe it is merely a surfacing of people who were already there – and who now stand up to be counted after the major social change that occurred as a result of the Stone Wall riots in New York City.

But I have a different theory. And while this remains unproven theory, I believe it will nevertheless provide a very insightful view into the entire condition concerning the relations between women and men as they exist today.

My observation is that the Women's Movement that started in the 1960's was the great turning point in the relations between the sexes in our time. The origins of that movement were quite valid, such as equal pay for equal work and life options for women that meant more choices than being a teacher or a nurse or a homemaker.

But to achieve those worthwhile ends, the seeds of distrust between men and women were sown. To make things sharper, and as a means to bring clarity to the struggle, men were declared "evil" by a fair number of the leaders of the Women's Movement. Men were depicted as aligning themselves against women to prevent their progress. Men were "plotting" to keep women "enslaved." Indeed, it was a very black and white picture held up, with no room for shades of gray.

And so women came to believe through constant repetition of those themes that proper female behavior was to be suspicious of every move a man made – to never trust a man in the least.

Most men, of course, are not sitting around imagining and plotting such things. Time and study have shown that men have been as much a victim in their own way as women in the roles the sociological forces of society define for them through the gradual historical and cultural changes that shape the roles both sexes play at any moment in time.

But, in seeing that a time for change had arrived, and as the Women's Movement successfully took hold, the die was cast. It was seen by many women that the only way to completely throw off the "shackles" women bore was to make the message extreme. And so a wedge – if not a stake – was driven into the ability to trust that began separating men and women to the degree they have arrived at today. And instead of being a short way apart, which was the original hope for "equality" on the part of women, many men and women now feel the gulf between the sexes is miles and miles and miles in distance, even moreso than in the past.

And, unfortunately, those possessing that view regarding separation appear to be right. The gulf is enormous, as anyone trying to date today quickly realizes.

So one can understand – at least from the point of view of my theory – as to why and how we've created our own world of loneliness and have even been able to conclude that love no longer exists. How could there be anything else when virtually no one seems able to find the road map to cross what appears vast distances to get to love?

Let's apply a little more practical sense: People inherently need affection. People need to be touched and held. People need the joys of sex. People need to be wanted – and loved, if possible.

So, within today's circumstances, if one can't get such things from the opposite sex, how many choices are left? And how many are willing to go a whole lifetime living a celibate life just because they can't reach and break through to the opposite sex, and, indeed, may, under the terms described above, literally hate the opposite sex for what has happened between them? So it all gets very messy.

Thus, we are where we are today.

It is, therefore, my belief that many people are living lives that they would not be living under more "normal" circumstances. It is also my belief that – as the British have viewed it for so long in their boys' schools – that homosexuality may well be a transitional phase in learning how to relate – a simpler form of affection in that two people of the same sex obviously think rather closely alike – a stage that many people cannot get past today in moving to the more complex relationship that exists between men and women because of the mental and physical differences.

Do not make the mistake in thinking that I am sitting in judgment, or that I believe that people cannot reach a mature and loving state as homosexuals. They absolutely can, as many couples coming out into the open as the barriers fall regarding gay marriage clearly demonstrate. I suggest only that it appears to my observation that conditions today are such that many people whose development would be to move on to a heterosexual love are blocked and arrested in such progress because of the difficult barriers that have arisen between the sexes in contemporary times.

I suggest only that until such time as the general population has reached a level of acceptance that is truly humane and equitable regardless of one's particular sexual affinity, that in terms of achieving a lasting and fully rich love, the odds are still greater for long-term success on the side of a heterosexual relationship – however stacked the odds are against even that happening today. But dramatic change is occurring within our society, and the shift to a belief that one should have a right to love and happiness wherever one may be lucky enough to find it as the preeminent standard, rather than dictating a lifetime of misery and loneliness to others for the sake of one's own prejudice, appears to now be taking place.

And please do not forget that what this book is about is finding love, real love. It is not about the politics of sex, sexual preference, attempting to change social trends, or any other subject. Those are very great and complex issues, and far too much to be dealt with here. The issue of love itself is huge enough in and of itself.

And though, as I observed at the outset of this chapter, monumental love is absolutely possible within a homosexual love, and it appears that the psychology of homosexual love does, in large part, very much follow the development of love in heterosexuals, the fact still remains that in our day and age, as the turmoil over gay marriage demonstrates, we are still dealing with both gay culture and gay love as a work in progress.

That being so, the current circumstances also speak to true courage on the part of those who pursue real love within such difficult boundaries, and, doubtless, as love will always do, there will be those who find love against such odds, as more and more are demonstrating is true through their declaration of love through marriage.

One day, the pendulum will swing, as it has done continually throughout history, and the current objections will perhaps no longer be an issue and be replaced by a more humane view of human happiness as the foremost of human objectives, but when that will happen, no one can currently foresee… Your own thoughts and opinions on this matter – whichever way they fall – surely demonstrate that is true. But homosexual love does exist, and we'd be foolish to pretend that it does not.

♥

Equal to the gods seems to me that man who sits facing you
And hears you nearby
Sweetly speaking and softly laughing.
This sets my heart to fluttering in my breast,
For when I look on you a moment,
Then can I speak no more,
But my tongue falls silent,
And at once a delicate flame courses beneath my skin,
And with my eyes I see nothing,
And my ears hum,
And a cold sweat bathes me,
And a trembling seizes me all over,
And I am paler than grass,
And I feel that I am near to death.

– SAPPHO
*Fragment 2*

# 11. CAN LOVE SURVIVE?

♥ That is really a foolish question. The immediate answer is: "Love WILL survive." The real distinguishment I'm trying to make is that love – at least in our time, unless there's a major shift in attitude – will, I believe, be a minimalist affair, maintained and carried on by those who, in the main, discover love accidentally.

The portrait I am painting is that of a tragedy. Many, many people will, I am afraid, date, marry, have sex, have children and raise a family together – and live out their lives as strangers, never having the slightest idea of what true intimacy and love could mean. The greater tragedy is that what I'm saying almost assuredly will be true for large numbers of people in our population.

Such a statement – one that may seem like a challenge to many people's way of life – is enough, I am sure, to make many want to rise up and condemn me.

But make no mistake, I'm really not condemning a soul for living their life as they choose. The truth is that many are fine with the arrangement of life as it is commonly played out today. Companionship is more than enough for many. Wild sex is actually not a requirement for the vast majority, in fact (other than in fantasy perhaps).

A "normal" existence like one's neighbors have can yield contentment. And if people find satisfaction in such a life, that's wonderful, in my estimation. Satisfaction, happiness, is – after all – the entire point of life, and there are as many definitions of happiness as there probably are people.

What I am really attempting to describe is that there is a world heaped with treasure if one is willing to strive for more, but most, thanks to the way we are educated regarding love today, don't even know that might be true. But, once one is aware of it, the amazing fact is that one can possess a life full of love whether one is a retail clerk or a millionaire.

And, perhaps, if you're already married and you happened to have happened upon this book and read it, maybe you'll find that it's time to take the time to fall in love with your mate. It's really all a matter of learning to trust completely and using good communication. Great love is not limited to the stunning redhead at the office or the handsome movie star. It is available to us all.

But most just don't know how to go about finding it. Now you do.

As to the fate of love, you and I will pass away one day, but love will endure forever. You need not fear for its safety. Right now we live in a world where the great cycles of life have brought love to a very lowly and degraded state, so low that many suggest it is only a concept that really doesn't exist. But, you may be sure, it is still here. There are those carrying the torch forward on behalf of all of us, however invisible they may be to the rest of the world, whether we appreciate that fact or not.

If I have one wish for you, it is that you become one of those able to step through that magic door into that parallel universe filled with light and joy. Then it will be your discovery, and your turn to say, "The greatest thing you'll ever learn is just to love and be loved in return."

Perhaps this little book will serve as the beginning of the pendulum swinging back the other way, as the word begins to spread that love is real and does exist. Perhaps we'll realize it's time to teach our children about the importance of love in human life and to begin guiding them so they can reach this full and happy stage of human existence as a natural part of life, rather than each generation simply letting the next stumble blindly forward as has happened for so long now, hoping that by accident our children will find love. Doesn't the former approach – giving young people the "roadmap" for finding love – seem a lot better than the latter? In any case, it's certainly worth thinking about.

# 12. IS THERE ANYTHING MORE ONE CAN SAY?

♥ John Lennon and Paul McCartney were great geniuses of the love song. The Beatles' albums are full of remarkable insight and commentary on the nature of love, which was central to all of their work, and their timeless songs never grow old or dated.

But what appears to me to be the most profound statement that came out of their work was a message as true and deep and simple as that of the poetry of Eden Abhez 's "Nature Boy," when they sang in the song "The End" that "the love you take is equal to the love you make."*

Understand that and you will always truly understand love.

♥

* John Lennon & Paul McCartney, "The End," *Abbey Road*, Northern Songs, 1969.

♥

# 13. A BOOK TO READ AND SOME MOVIES TO SEE

♥There are certainly many books and movies – as well as other resources – one might refer to in the exploration of love. The following are four contemporary recommendations, which I believe can be of real value to those who will take the time to experience them.

**LIVING WELL IS THE BEST REVENGE** by Calvin Tomkins
New York: The Viking Press, 1971

This little book is a portrait of a very great and admirable love – that of Sara and Gerald Murphy. Readers will find that many of the characteristics of love as I have described them are clearly apparent in the lives of these two individuals who truly became one. I am a strong believer in role models – heroes and heroines, if you will – and you will find the Murphy's love is an excellent example to hold up before you. If they could achieve a great love, so can you.

*Living Well Is the Best Revenge* first appeared as an article in *The New Yorker* magazine in 1962, and was later issued in book form.

**GOODBYE, MR. CHIPS**
The musical motion picture starring Peter O'Toole and Petula Clark, 1969

This very great motion picture remains to this day extremely unappreciated. The score by Leslie Bricusse is, in fact, one of the finest and most poetic ever created for a motion picture. This classic story of the love between a school master at an English boy's school and a London musical theatre star is virtually an instruction book on the nature of give and take that occurs in a great love, and the feelings that are involved. Again, this is an extraordinary role model example for people to study.

**BROKEBACK MOUNTAIN**
The motion picture starring Heath Ledger and Jake Gyllenhaal, 2005

Based upon the short story by Annie Proulx, this film masterpiece not only brilliantly depicts the complexity of the issues faced by homosexual love, but it also captures the emotions of the nature of true love, demonstrating how love transcends all boundaries which humans may apply in trying to contain it.

**THE NOTEBOOK**
The motion picture starring Ryan Gosling and Rachel McAdams, 2004

A film that captures the character and many of the rich emotions of true love. This film is almost astonishing in its power to depict love and what it can be.

# *ACKNOWLEDGEMENTS*

I very much appreciate the kindness of David J. Janowiak, Golden World Music, publisher of Eden Abhez's "Nature Boy," for permitting me to reproduce Mr. Abhez's extraordinary lyrics/ poetry.

I would also like to thank the Reverend Bryant Wright, Senior Pastor of Johnson Ferry Baptist Church, Marietta, Georgia, for the use of his wise and humane radio broadcast texts from his Right From The Heart Ministries (www.rfth.org), which have made a difference in my own life.

This is a personal essay, therefore, it is personal opinion. The kindness of these two gentlemen in allowing me to share the above-indicated ideas with readers does not constitute agreement nor endorsement on their part with all I say. But we do agree on one point: We all believe in the power of love. I hope you do, as well.


*James R. Messenger*
Marietta, Georgia, USA

♥

JAMES R. MESSENGER is a graduate of both the University of Georgia (A.B.J., 1970) and Georgia State University (M.B.A., 1994).

He is the author of the books *Excuse Me, Please, But I'd Like My Government Back* and *The Death of the American Telephone & Telegraph Company – How "Ma Bell" Died Giving Birth to the Information Age*.

He has written for a wide spectrum of print publications, ranging from *Reader's Digest* to *American Cinematographer* to *New Jersey English Journal* to *The Atlanta Journal-Constitution* and *The Marietta Daily Journal.*

Among many awards, Jim Messenger has won an EMMY for his film "The Taj Mahal," a film about one of history's great love stories, and he has also been nominated twice for Academy Awards for "OF TIME, TOMBS AND TREASURE: The Treasures of Tutankhamun" and "Koryo Celadon."

He also traveled 18,000 miles across the United States and looked upon the faces of an estimated 30-50,000,000 Americans in making his documentary film, "CARRY THE FIRE: The Story of the 1984 Olympic Torch Relay."

In the business sphere, he has twice won the prestigious "Corporate Identity Award" from the Public Relations Society of America for AT&T and EXXON Corporation.

On December 12, 1982, Jim Messenger conceived the Theory of the Information Age, which has proven to be his most enduring contribution to society.

Printed in the United States
123269LV00001B/25-30/P